A GUIDE TO PRE AND POST NATAL EXERCISE

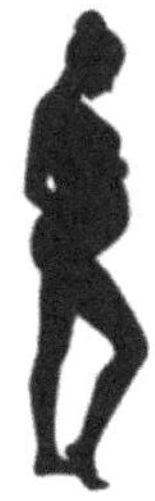

CONTENTS

INTRODUCTION

The Author

Barrie Beattie is an Exercise Therapist, Personal Trainer, Performance Nutritionist and Fitness Instructor with well over a decade of experience in the fitness industry. He first fell in love with training 20 years ago as a teenager and has helped hundreds of people reach their fitness and lifestyle goals. He is also a competitive bodybuilder and has represented Great Britain in his sport.

Why I chose to write this book...

There are many reasons for me choosing to write a manual on pre- and post-natal exercise. It is not a topic which generally befits a male personal trainer especially from a bodybuilding background. But over the past 4 years or so I have noticed distinct flaws in the information being given out to mothers when returning to work or more rather the lack of information being given. People scare mongering that you must not do exercise if you are pregnant or planning to get pregnant. Then there is the complete opposite end of the scale that you can and should be doing copious amount of weight training or go out pounding the pavements by running endless miles.

There are clinicians actively telling people the best exercise for the pelvic floor post birth is stopping yourself from peeing mid flow, by the way this is not the best pelvic floor exercise or even an exercise at all. Something as simple as a brief chat with an exercise therapist or physiotherapist who knows what they are talking about and a well-constructed programme would be sufficient to give all mothers a point in the right direction. This book will provide the information needed in an easy-to-use format with pictures for demonstration.

All the exercises and techniques detailed within this book have been tried and tested and are currently being used by clinicians and physical trainers as pre- and post-natal treatment for women. I have used the exact same techniques for my own wife after she gave birth to our child and she found them extremely beneficial as have several personal training clients. This book is not designed to be an exhaustive manual that you must follow from start to finish. It is a guide you can try at home or at work. Within this guide there are exercises that are pitched at the correct level with appropriate progressions and regressions.

Benefits of Exercise Before and During Pregnancy

- Quicker recovery post-natal.
- Reduced maternal weight.
- Reduced swelling.
- Improved circulation.
- Can help prevent high blood pressure.

CHAPTER 1 – THE EFFECTS OF PREGNANCY ON THE BODY

There are many effects on the human body during pregnancy. These effects involve the muscular skeletal system, the cardiovascular system, the respiratory system, and the hormones in your body.

During pregnancy there will be laxity at the structures surrounding your joints. This laxity will put you at a greater risk of injuries, so this is something to keep in mind when exercising or performing manual tasks. This does not mean you cannot exercise however be mindful.

The main thing which is going to cause changes to your body during pregnancy is the hormones being produced. These hormones include Progesterone, Oestrogen and Relaxin. These hormones effect the body as follows.

Progesterone

Causes a reduction in smooth muscle mass, an increase in body temperature by 0.5 – 1 Degree Centigrade, possible hyperventilation, increased fat storage and a reduction of alveolar and arterial PCO2 (Partial Pressure of Carbon Dioxide) which is the effectiveness of ventilation in the lung's alveoli (air sacks). This is a good indicator of respiratory function.

Oestrogen

Oestrogen is a hormone which promotes and maintains female characteristics of the body. Oestrogen production causes increased water retention which would also result in weight gain.

Relaxin

Relaxin starts to be produced 2 weeks into gestation (the period of foetal development in the womb between conception and birth). This is the hormone which causes laxity or loosening of the structures around the joints. It can take up to 5 months post pregnancy for joint structures to stabilise due to relaxin being produced (NCT 2018).

Cardiovascular System

The cardiovascular (CV) system is made up of the heart, lungs and blood vessels. During pregnancy, the heart size can increase with a 30-50% increase in cardiac output (the amount of blood pumped by the heart in a minute), this will result in a small rise in heart rate. Haemoglobin (protein that transports oxygen around your body in blood) levels may fall to 80% of what they usually are.

Respiratory System

You may notice symptoms of nasal congestion due to swelling of the lining of the nose, oropharynx, larynx and trachea. Oxygen consumption also increases due to the needs of the growing foetus. (Mother & Child Glossary, 2002)

Muscular Skeletal System

Due to relaxin being released from the beginning of the pregnancy, which helps enable the pelvis to expand during the birth by increasing the laxity (looseness) in the ligaments around the pelvis. Other effects of relaxin also include increased mobility in joints such as the hips and those of the feet. This starts to show at 6 weeks, and peak at 12 weeks. This can lead to pain around the pelvis and lower back. Other joints of the body are also affected, and the laxity can cause hypermobility (excessive movement) and this puts the person at an increased risk of injury and the persons biomechanics will also be affected.

The muscles of the abdomen are stretched during pregnancy causing a loss of strength within this area. Diastasis recti (a split of the linea alba ligament in the centre of the abdominals) will also occur and will need to be considered when exercising post birth. There will also be difficulty in maintaining neutral spine position due to growing abdomen, this will cause tightness in the hip flexors also tightness and possible pain in the lower back. Pain in the front of the pelvis is also normal.

CHAPTER 2 – WARMING UP AND STRETCHING DURING PREGNANCY

Warm up

It is always essential to warm the body up before exercise for a total of 10-15 minutes. For some this as simple as walking for 5 minutes before to warm the core temperature of the body followed by mobilisation and dynamic stretching (moving stretches) of the body parts you will be working is sufficient. Extra precautions should be taken with mothers expecting twins or who have become pregnant through IVF. Consult your doctor before commencing exercise. Some basic joint mobilisations to warm up are shown below, complete 12 to 30 repetitions whilst moving the joint passively (without squeezing the muscles).

Mobility

Shoulder Mobility

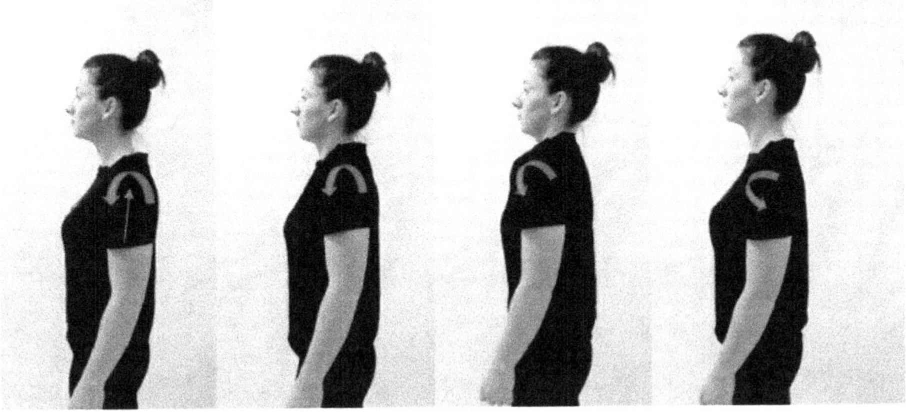

Spinal Mobility

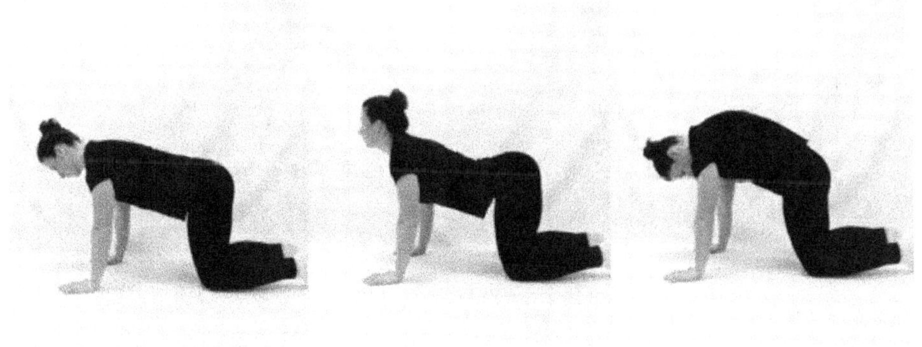

Spinal Mobility Continued...

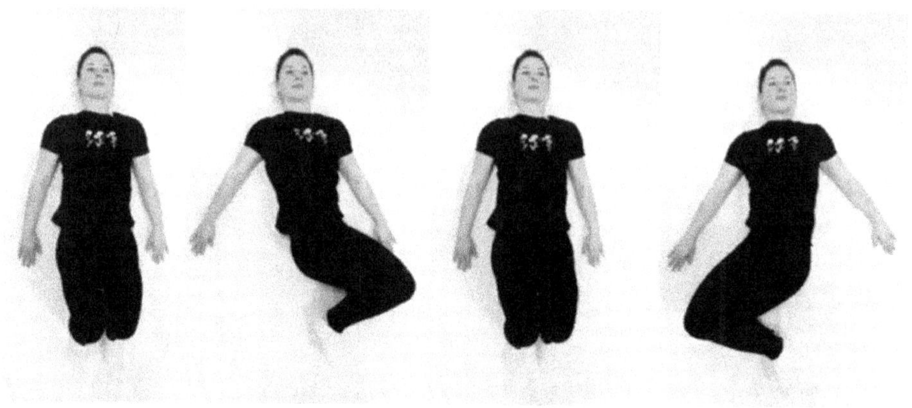

Hip Mobility

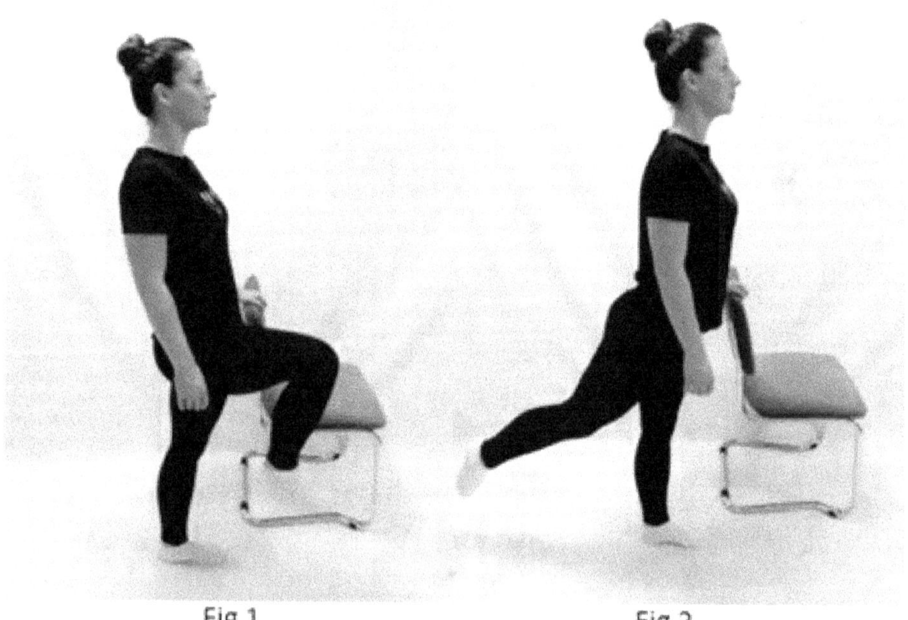

Fig 1   Fig 2

Hip Mobility Continued...

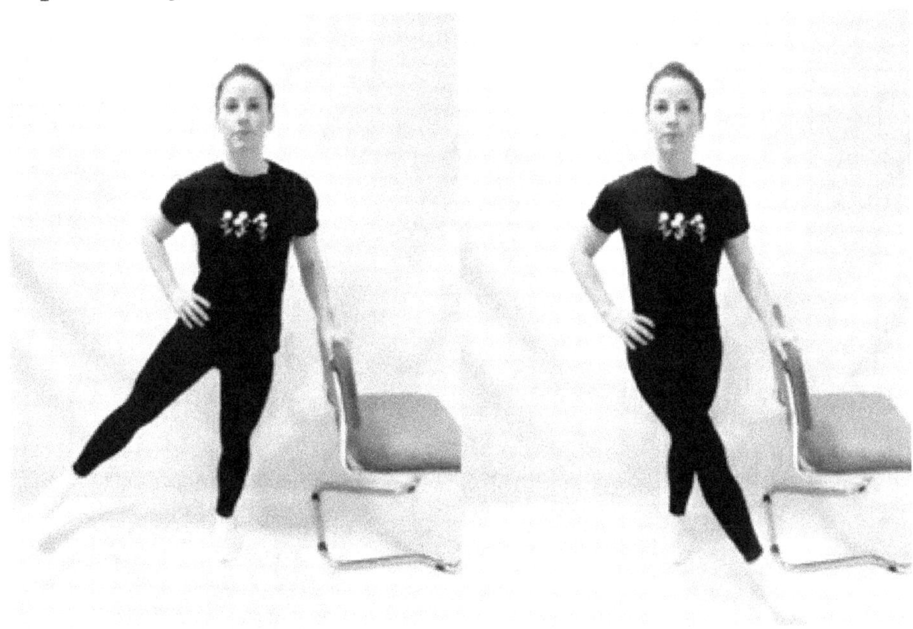

Fig 3   Fig 4

Knee Mobility

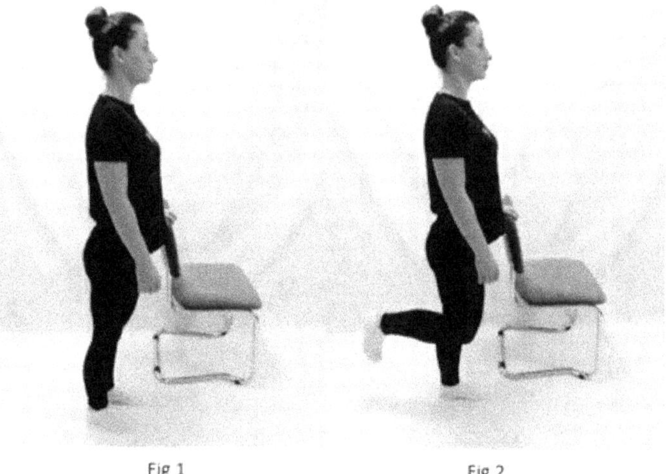

Fig 1   Fig 2

Ankle Mobility

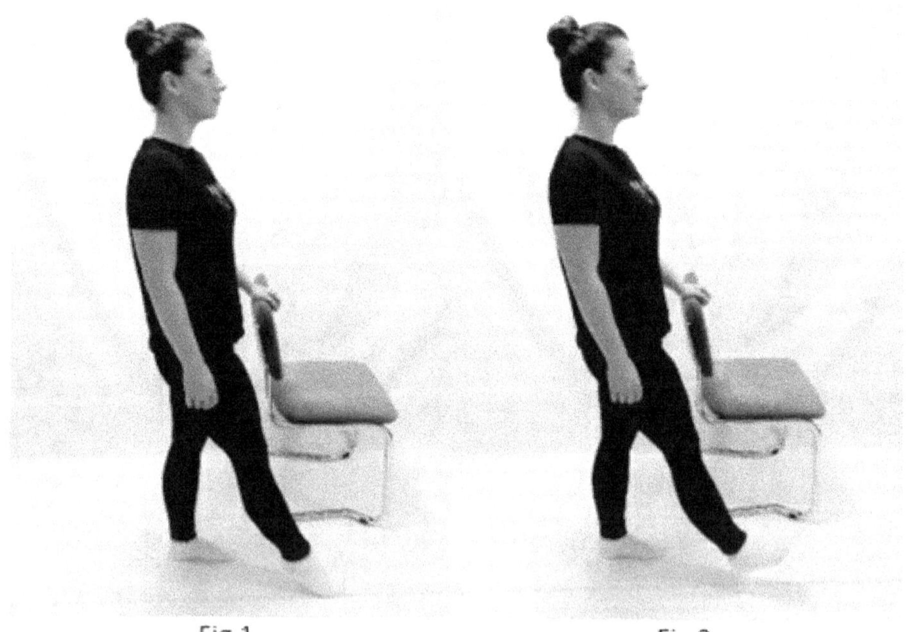

Fig 1   Fig 2

Pelvic Alignment

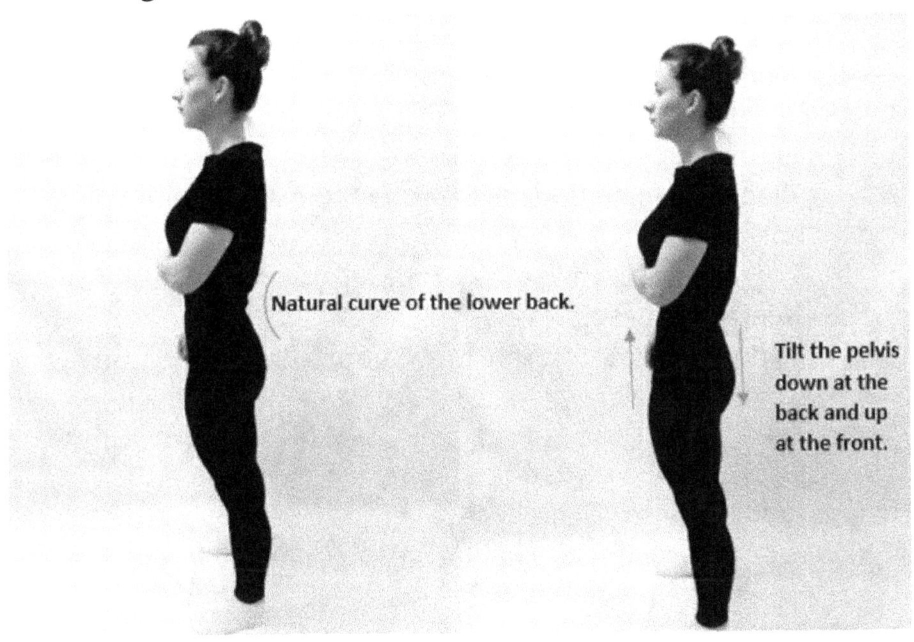

Stretches

Developmental stretches should be avoided due to joint laxity, therefore hold each stretch for a maximum of 30 seconds.

Chair Stretch

- Place a cushion on the floor in front of a couch or chair, kneel on the cushion and put the foot of the same leg on the chair.
- Place the other foot flat on the floor with a bend in your knee.
- Try to tense the buttock of the leg you are kneeling on.
- Keep your pelvis level.
- To decrease the stretch, move your knee further out away from the chair.

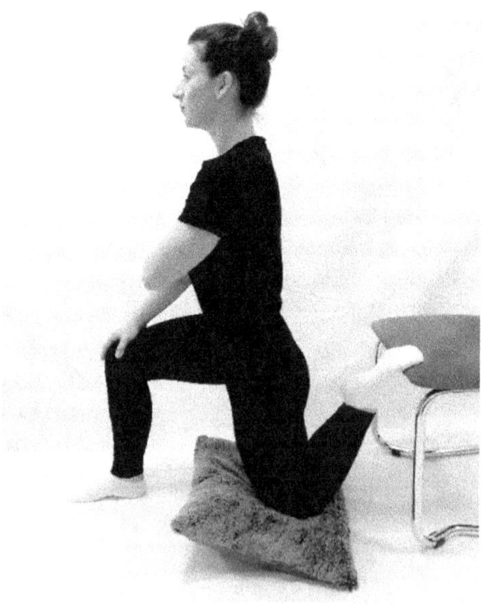

Kneeling Hip Flexor Stretch
- Same as previous, however the foot of the leg you are kneeling on should remain straight on the floor.

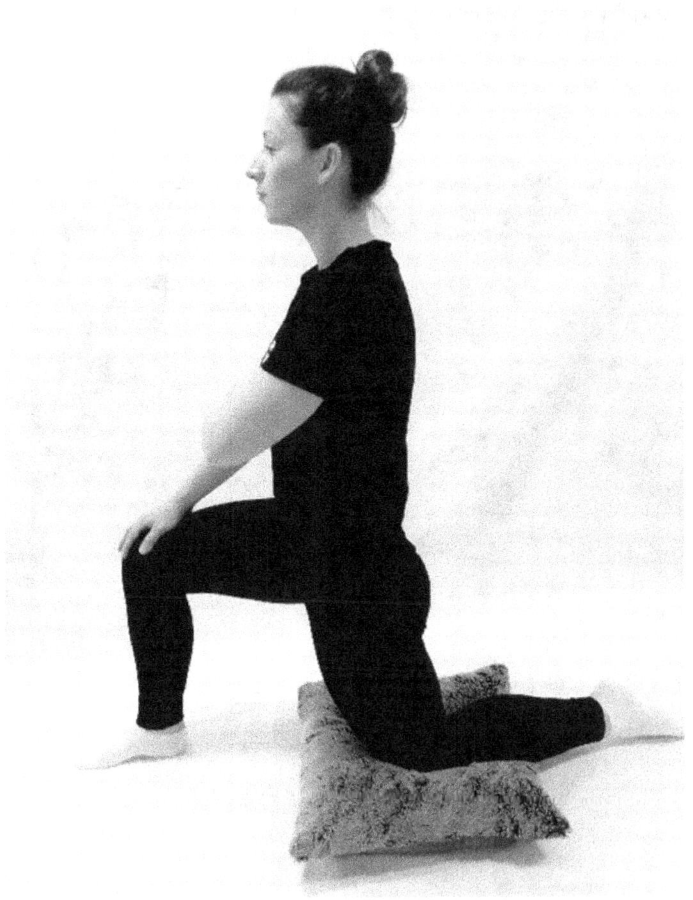

Lying TFL (Tensor Fasciae Latae) Stretch

- Lay flat on your back and bend one knee to 90 degrees.
- Place your bent leg at a 45 degrees angle to the body and allow the knee to drop in towards your other leg keeping your foot on the floor.
- Stand up between each stretch.

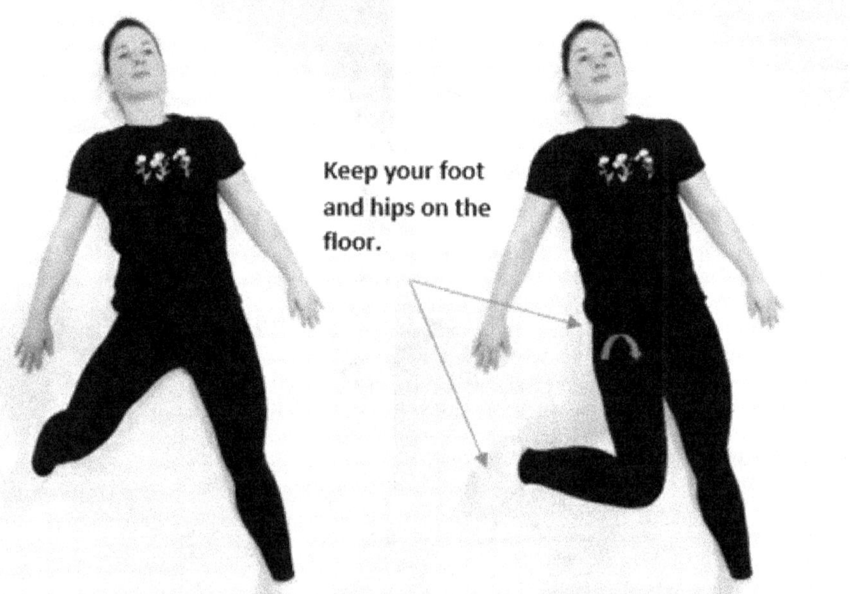

Lying TFL (Tensor Fasciae Latae) Stretch Continued...

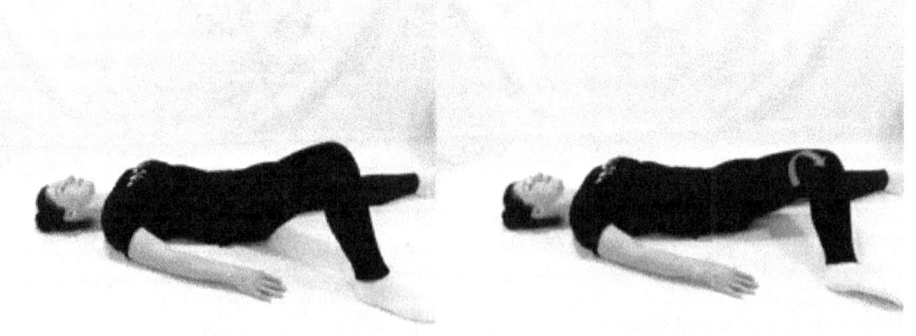

Seated Buttock Stretch (As able to)

- Sit on the floor with your legs straight out in front of you and place one of your feet over the other leg. Pull this leg in towards your body. You should feel this stretch in your buttock.

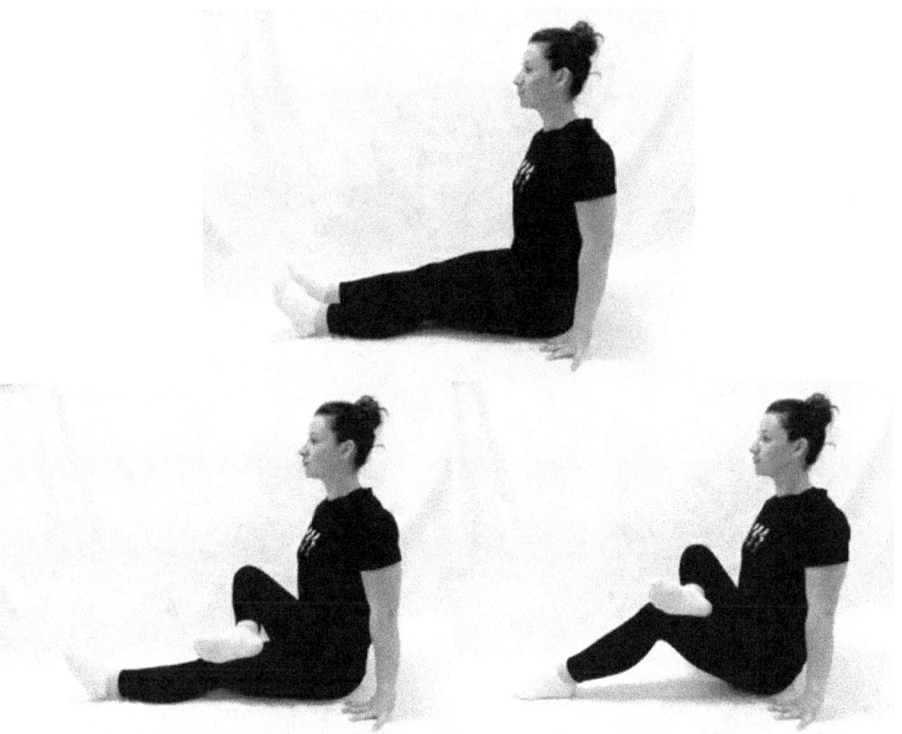

Pigeon Stretch (As able to)

- Go onto your knees on a comfortable surface like a carpet.
- Place one leg in front of the other, with your foot in front of your other knee and the outer part of your lower leg flat on the floor.
- Push your buttocks back until you feel a stretch.

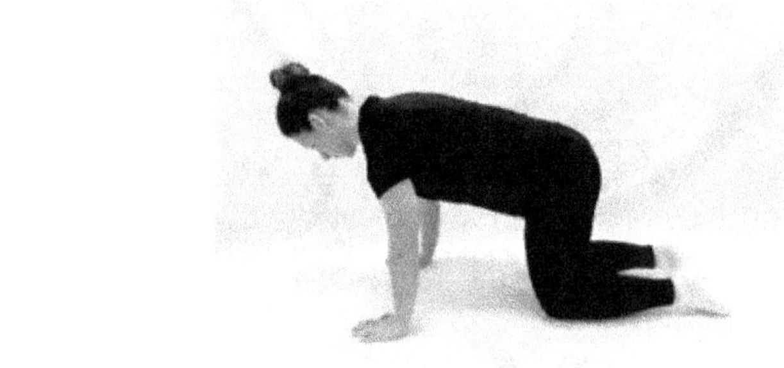

Fig 1

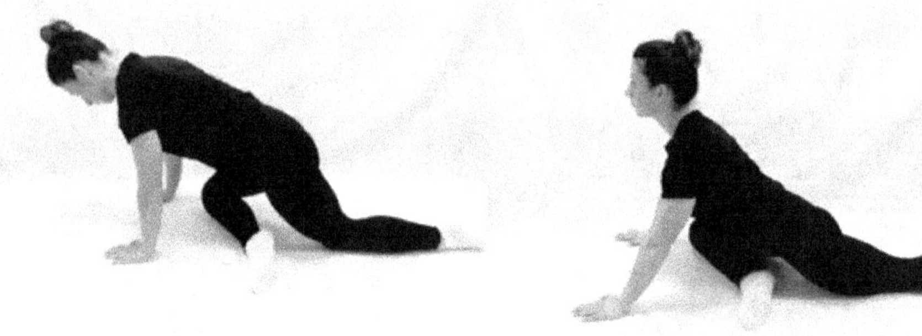

Fig 2

Fig 3

Standing Hamstring Stretch

- Stand with one foot in front of the other and bend your back leg.
- Have a slight bend in the leg in front at the knee, keep both your feet flat on the floor and look straight ahead.
- Push your buttocks back until you feel a stretch on the back of your thigh. Your hips (pelvis) should remain in line.

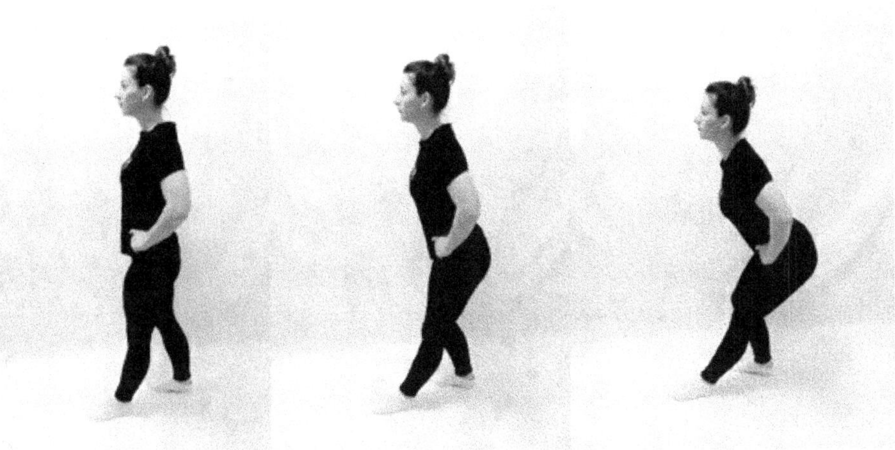

Standing Calf Stretch

-   Stand on a step or rolled up towel on one leg with your heel over the edge, hold onto the banister or a chair for support.
- Allow your heel to drop down until you feel a stretch in the back of your lower leg.
- To move the stretch further down put a slight bend in your knee. Your hips (pelvis) should remain in line.

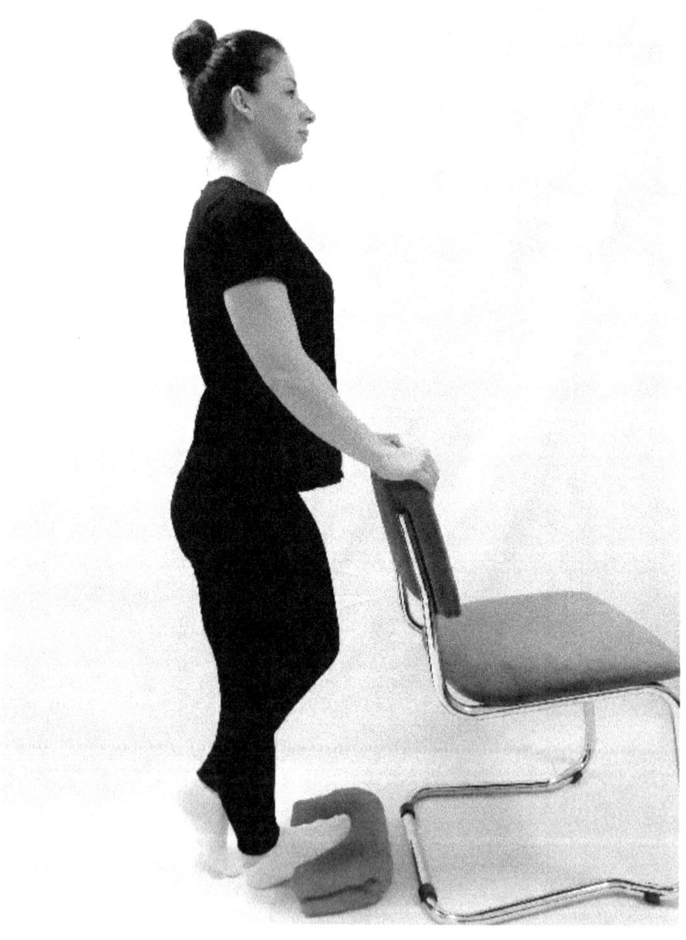

Standing Calf Stretch Continued...

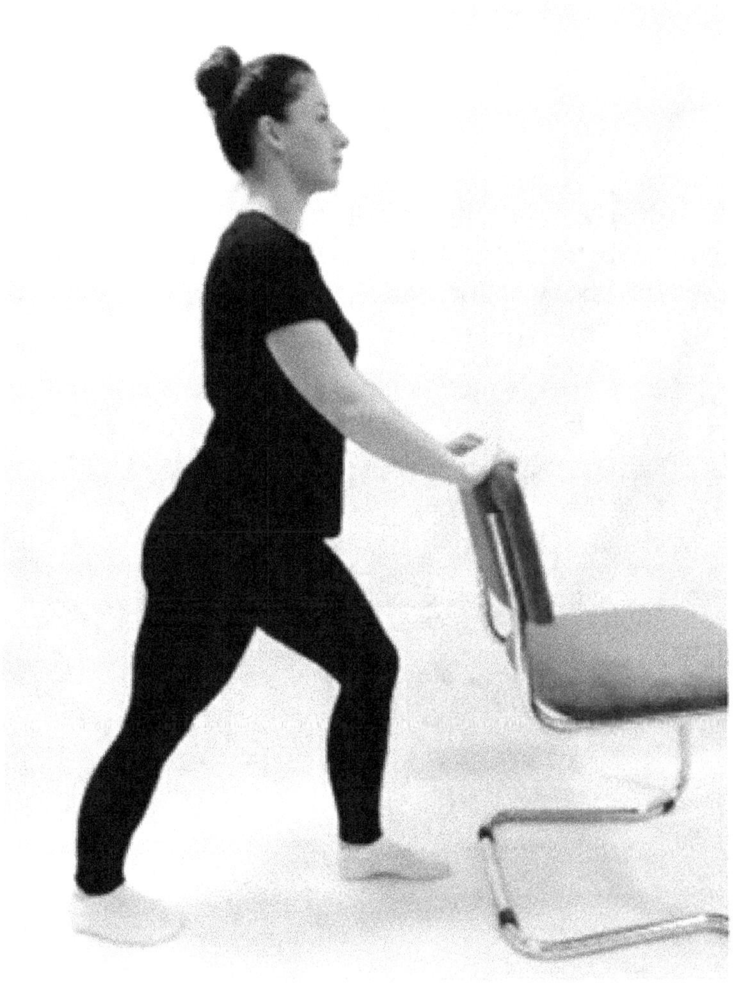

CHAPTER 3 – EXERCISES DURING PREGNANCY

During exercise you should avoid lying on your back (supine). Within your second trimester relaxin levels are at their highest therefore joint laxity is increased. Standing for long periods of time should also be avoided.

Tools

Dumbbells

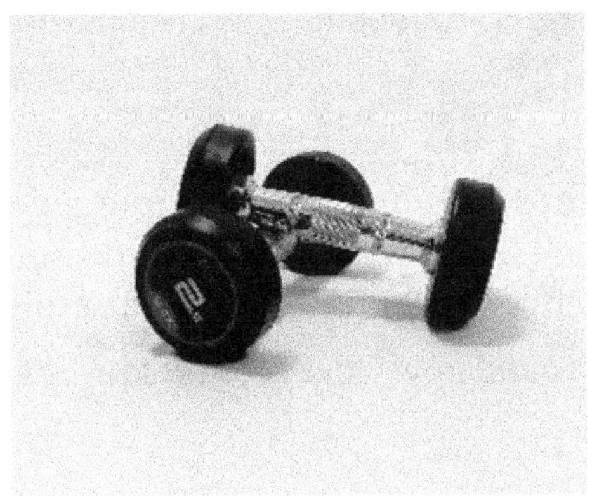

Resistance Band

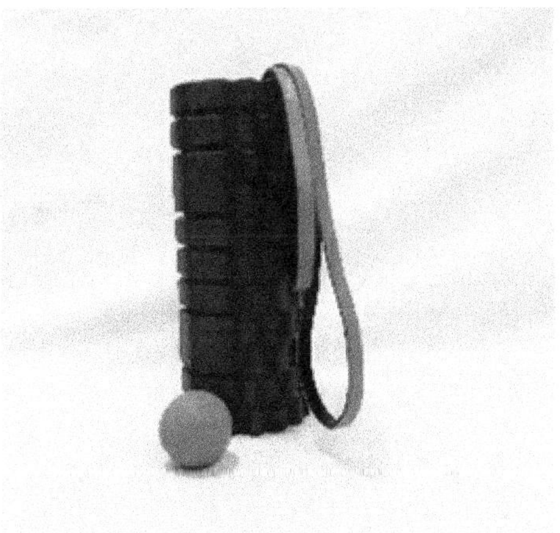

Repetitions

All exercises should be done for 3 lots of 15 repetitions on each side. Unless otherwise specified. Exercises can be done daily or as fatigue allows.

Tempo

Tempo is the speed at which you complete a repetition. It is broken down into three parts. The upwards, squeeze and downwards phases. Each of these phases is timed as follows:

1-2-2 means a 1 second upward-2 second squeeze-2 second downward.

Standing Hip Abduction

- Stand on one leg and hold onto something like a chair for support.
- Engage (tense) your abdominal muscles and bring your leg away and slightly back from your body at a 45 degrees angle.
- Ensure you are only moving at your hip joint and not at your waist.
- Squeeze the buttock of the leg you are moving and then slowly return to the start position.
- Tempo 1-2-2.

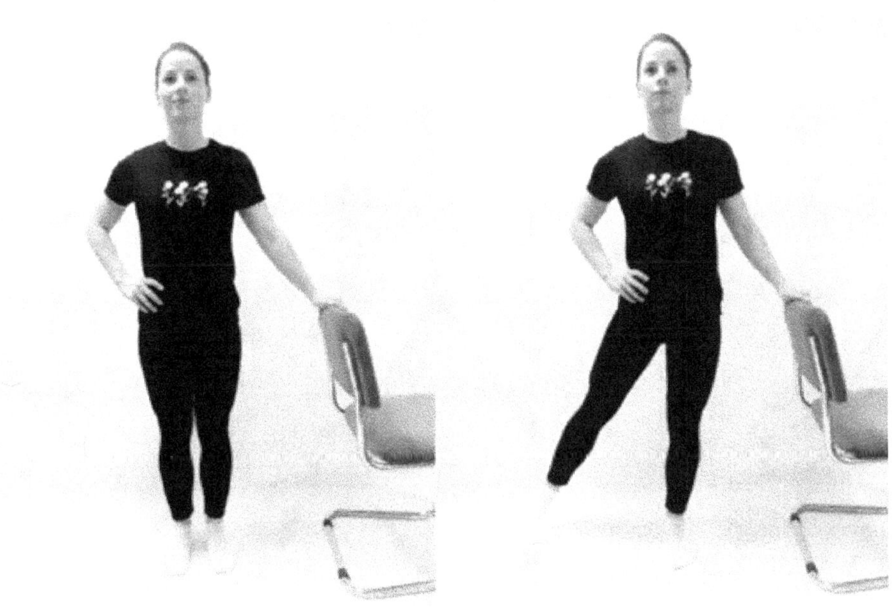

Kneeling Hip Extension

-   Kneel and hold onto something like a chair for support.
-   Engage (tense) your abdominal muscles and bring your leg directly back from your body.
-   Ensure you are only moving at your hip joint and not at your lower back.
-   Squeeze the buttock of the leg you are moving and then slowly return to the start position.
-   To make it more difficult lift the toes of the leg you are working off the floor when you are squeezing your buttock.
-   Tempo 1-2-2.

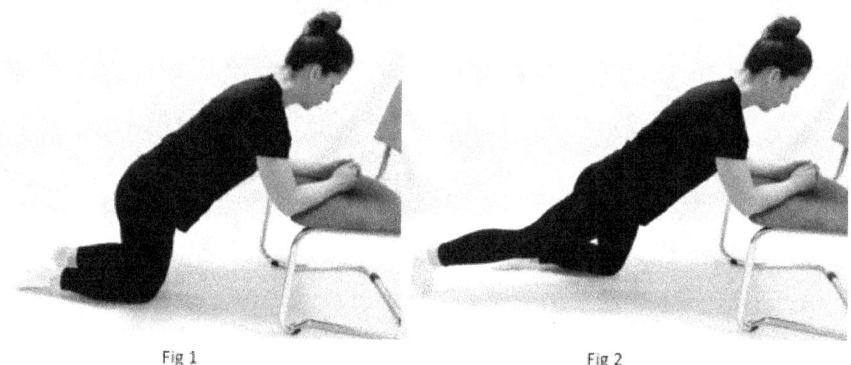

Fig 1   Fig 2

Chair Squats

- Place a chair behind you and stand with your feet in a natural and comfortable position.
- Slowly sit back onto the chair controlling the movement until you are fully seated.
- Stand back up without jerking your body forwards.
- Tense your buttocks as you begin to stand and move straight up (not forwards).
- Tempo 1-2-2.

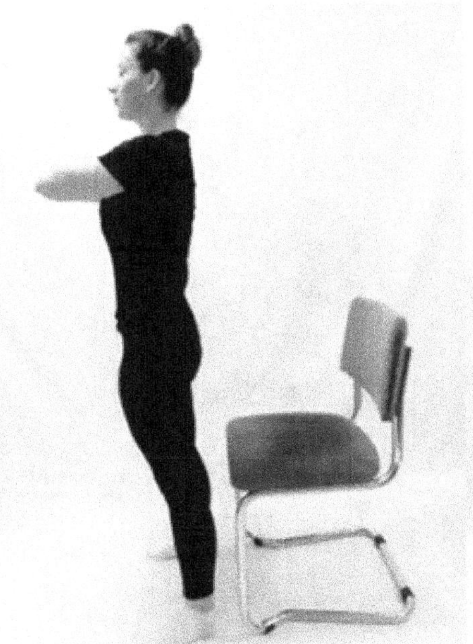

Fig 1

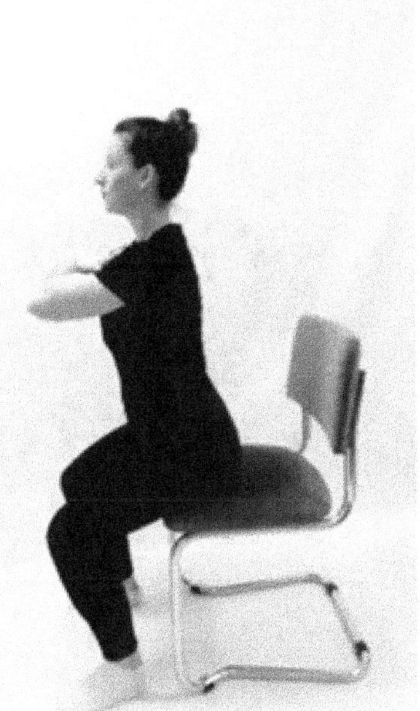

Fig 2

Side Plank

- Lay on one side on a comfortable surface with both knees bent at 90 degrees.
- Come up onto your forearm and your lower legs.
- Keep your knees and shoulders in line and maintain spinal alignment (see picture).
- Ensure your top shoulder over your bottom shoulder.
- Tempo N/A.
- Hold for a maximum of 30 seconds and repeat 2 – 3 times.

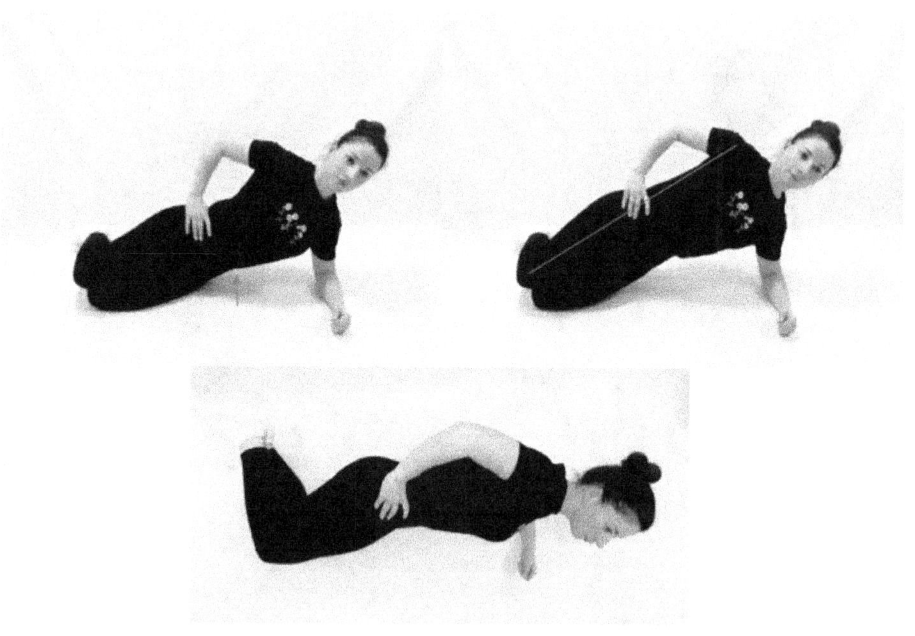

Clams

- Lie down on your side with both legs bent and your feet in line with your buttocks.
- Rest your head on your arm. Keep your free hand on your hip.
- Keeping your feet together slowly raise and lower your top knee.
- Your pelvis should remain in the same position through-out the movement and not move back and forth.
- Tempo 1-2-1.

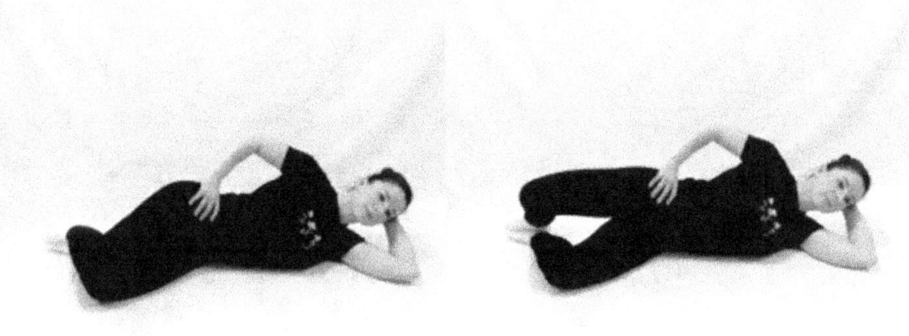

Fig 1   Fig 2

Feet Raised Clams

- Lie down on your side with both legs bent and your feet in line with your buttocks.
- Rest your head on your arm. Keep your free hand on your hip or the floor in front of you for balance.
- Raise both feet off the floor.
- Keeping your feet together slowly raise and lower your top knee.
- Your pelvis should remain in the same position throughout the movement and not move back and forth.
- Tempo 1-2-2.

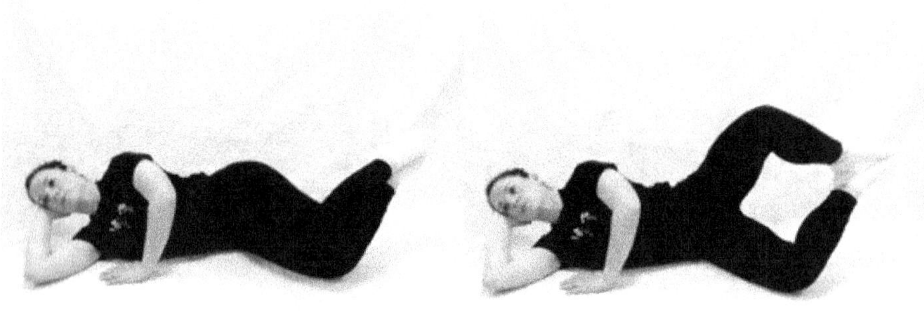

Fig 1   Fig 2

Hip Rotations

- Lie down on your side with both legs straight. Rest your head on your arm.
- Raise your upper leg and hold it in position.
- Rotate your hip forwards and backwards.
- Do up to 15 repetitions and repeat both side 3 times.
- Tempo 0.5-0.5-0.5.

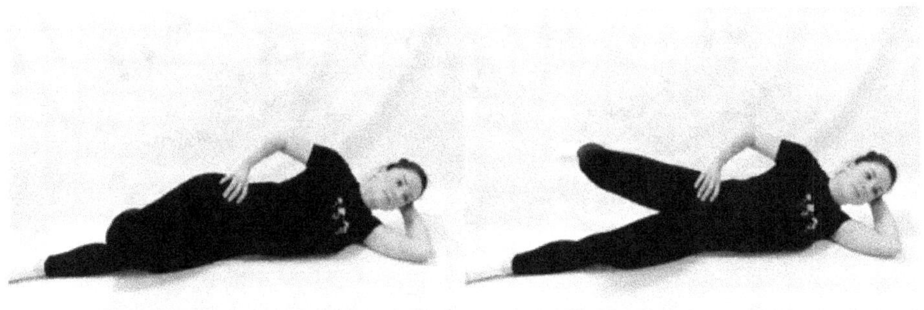

Fig 1   Fig 2

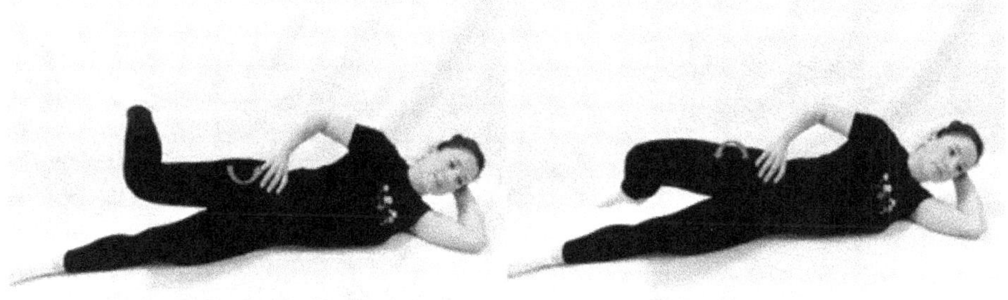

Fig 3   Fig 4

Hip Rotations Continued…

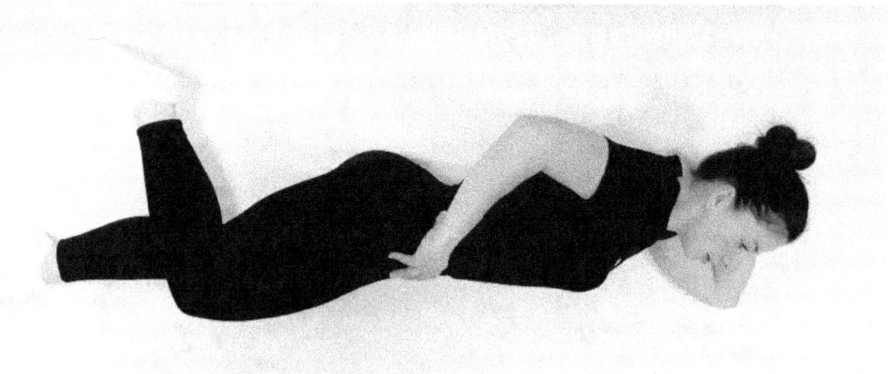

Fig 5

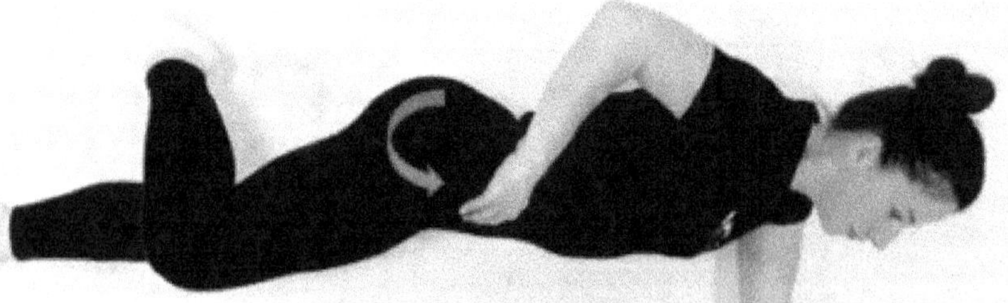

Fig 6

Toes raise off the floor and knees remain parallel.

Place your arm out in front of you to balance.

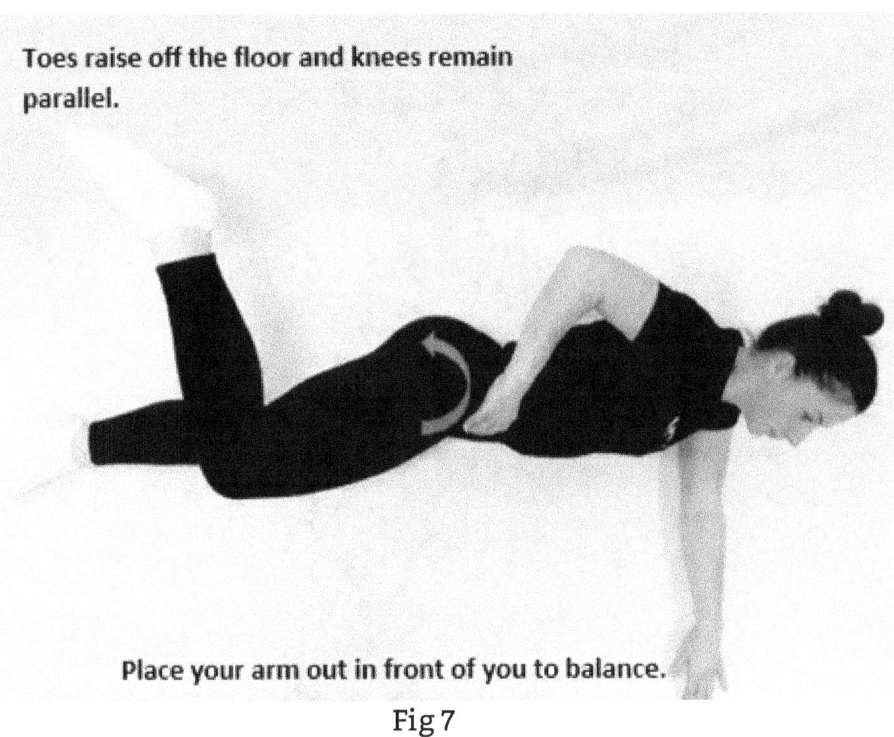

Fig 7

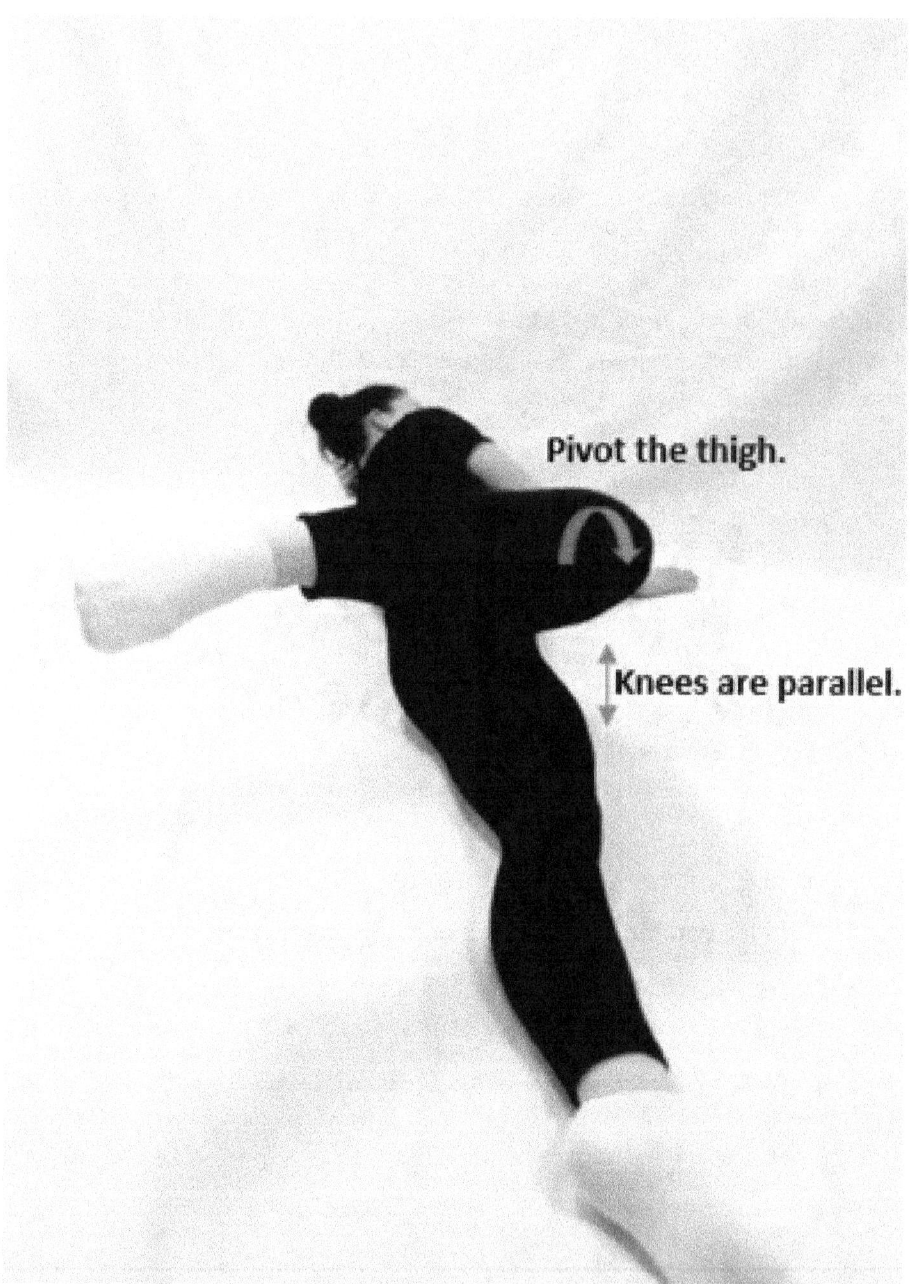
Pivot the thigh.
Knees are parallel.

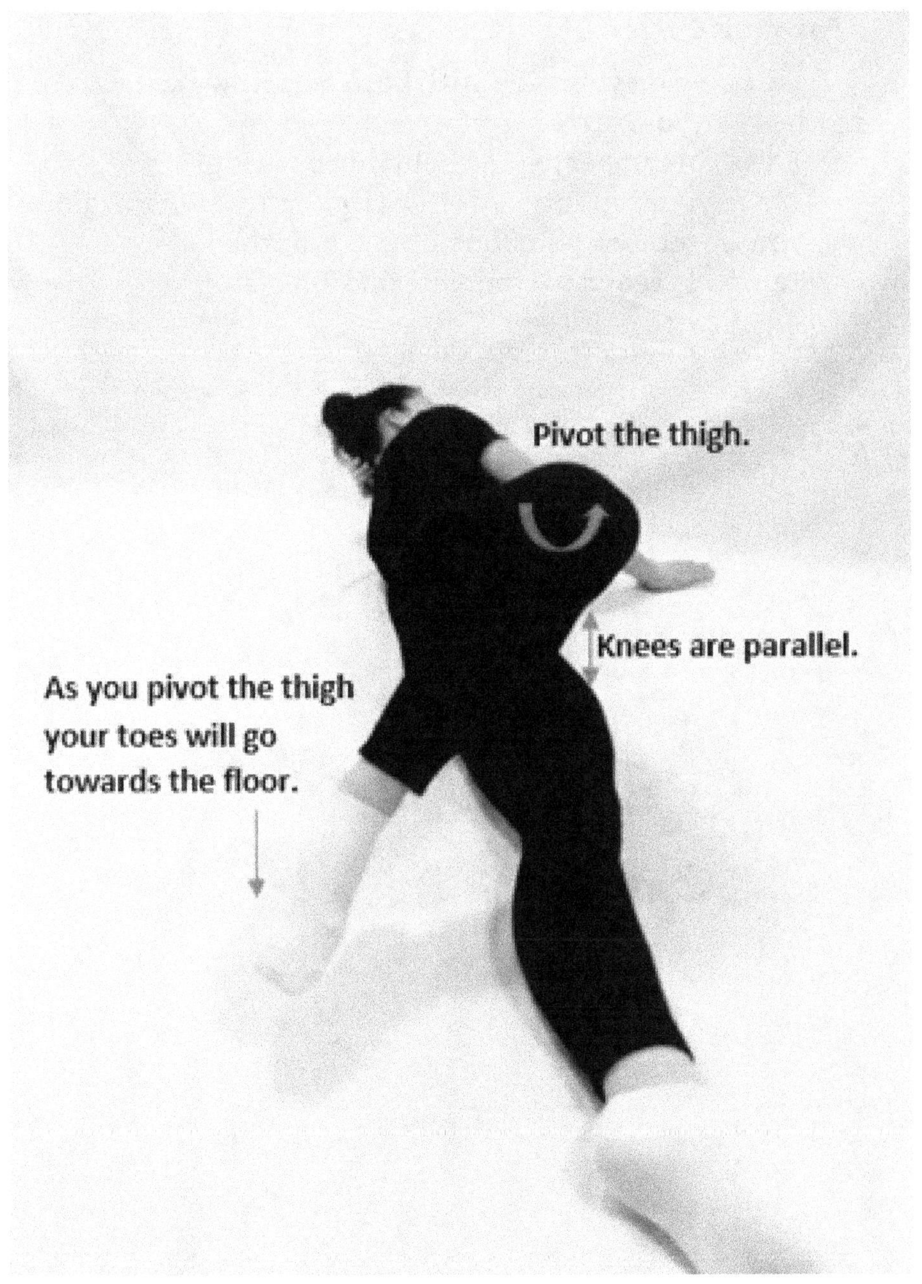
Pivot the thigh.
Knees are parallel.
As you pivot the thigh
your toes will go
towards the floor.

Forwards Circles

- Lie down on your side with both legs straight. Rest your head on your arm.
- Raise your upper leg and hold it in position.
- Move your hip forwards in a circular motion imagining you are moving your foot around a football.
- Tempo 1 second to complete one full circle.

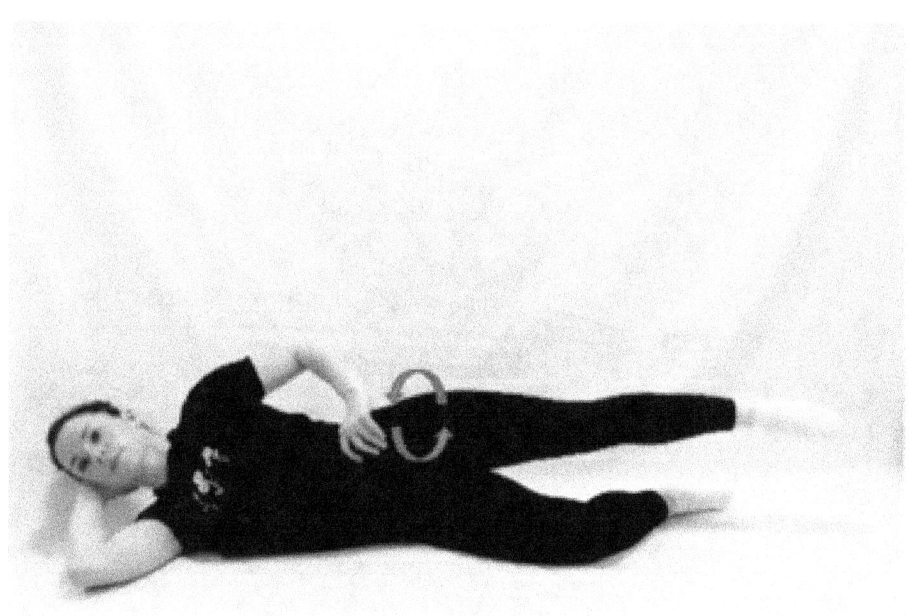

Side Lying Abduction

- Lie down on your side with both legs straight. Rest your head on your arm.
- Lift your upper leg up and slightly backwards, squeezing your bum and then slowly lower it.
- Tempo 1-2-2.

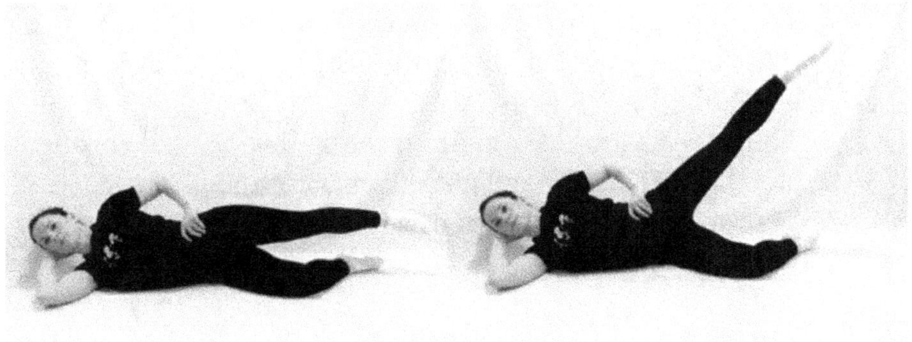

Fig 1   Fig 2

Running Man / Bicycle

- Lie down on your side with both legs bent and your feet in line with your buttocks. Rest your head on your arm. Keep your free hand on your hip.
- Keep your legs slightly apart.
- Keeping your bottom leg on the floor move your top leg in a running/cycling motion ensuring your legs remain parallel.
- Your pelvis should remain in the same position throughout the movement and not move back and forth.
- Tempo 2 to 3 seconds for one full repetition.

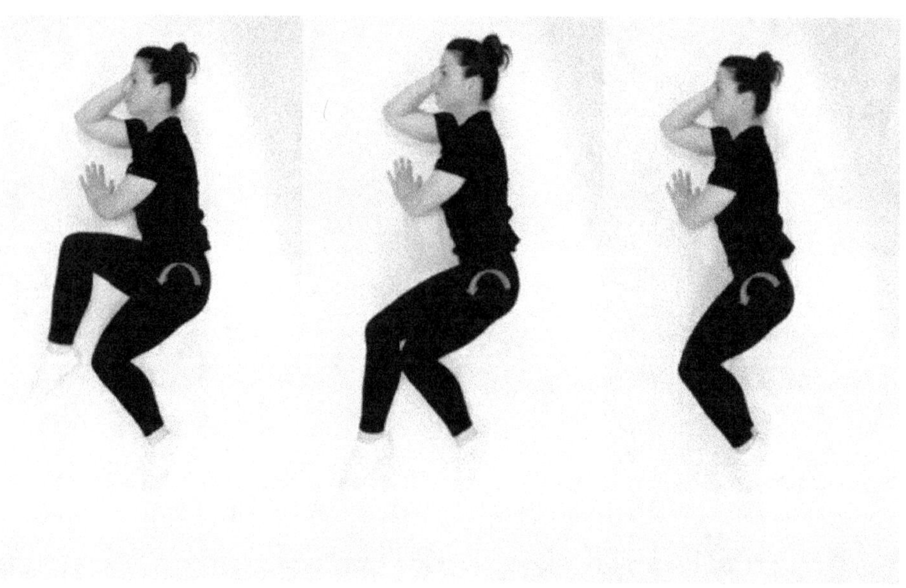

Fig 1

Running Man / Bicycle Continued...

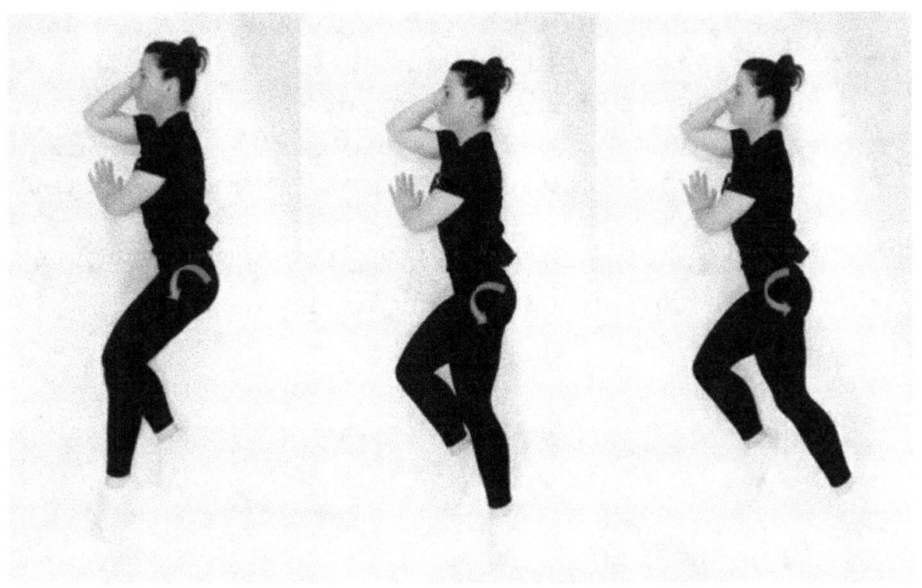

Fig 2

Straight Leg Clam

- Lie down on your side with your bottom leg straight and your top leg bent with your foot in line with your buttocks. Rest your head on your arm.
- Keep your free hand on your hip or on the floor in front of you.
- Keeping your foot on the floor slowly raise and lower your top knee.
- Your pelvis should remain in the same position throughout the movement and not move back and forth.
- Tempo 1-2-2.

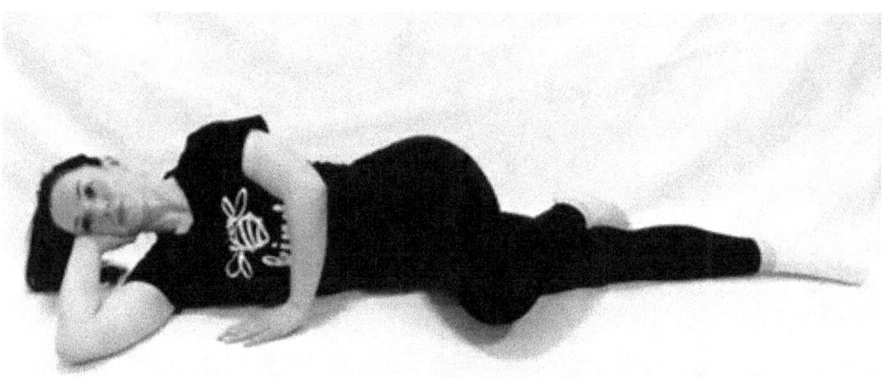

Fig 1

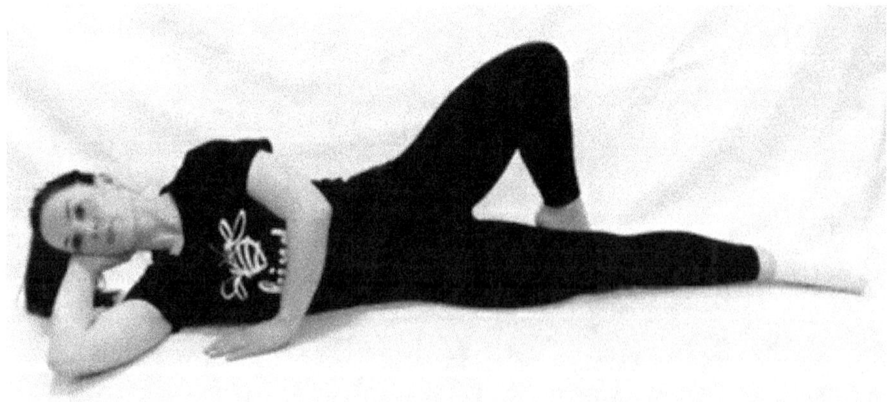

Fig 2

Straight Leg Clam continued...

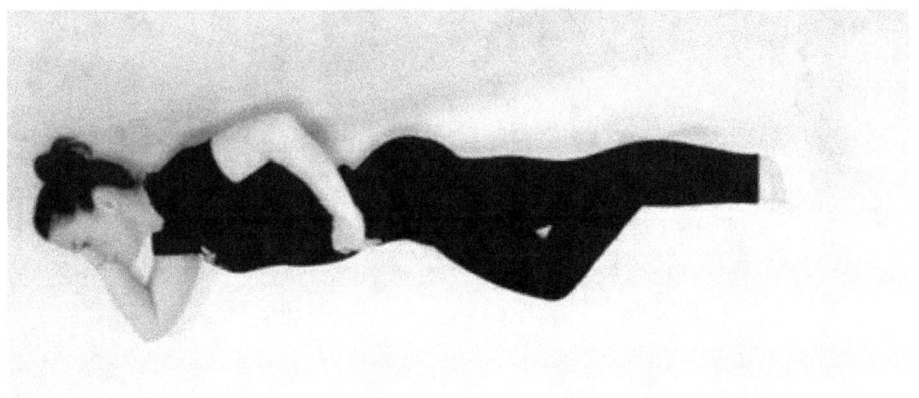

Fig 3

Standing Calf Raises

- Stand on the edge of a step or rolled up towel using a wall or chair for support.
- Gently lower your heels until you feel a stretch in your calf muscle.
- Push up keeping the weight through your pinkie toes.
- Tempo 1-2-2.

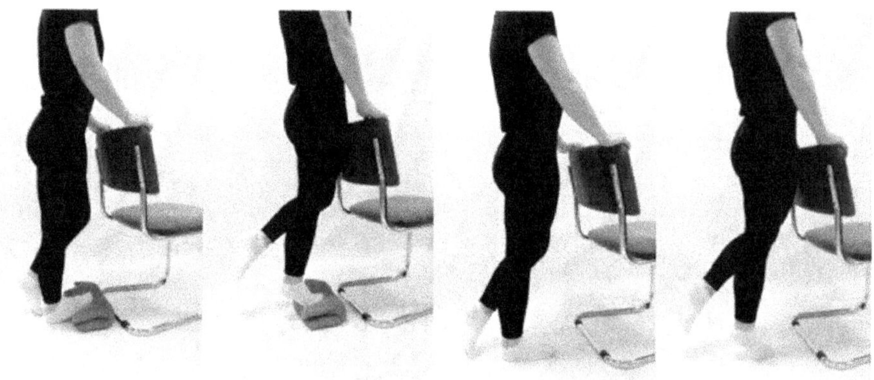

Fig 1   Fig 2

- Try doing this exercise on a flat surface to begin with if you find it difficult.

Seated Shoulder Press

- Sit on a chair with your feet on the floor just over shoulder width apart and your back straight, looking straight ahead.
- Start with your arms out to the sides with a 90degrees bend in the elbow.
- Raise your arms above your head until just before the elbows lock out and then slowly lower back to the start position.
- Use small weights or if you do not have any baked bean cans will do fine!
- Tempo 1-2-2.

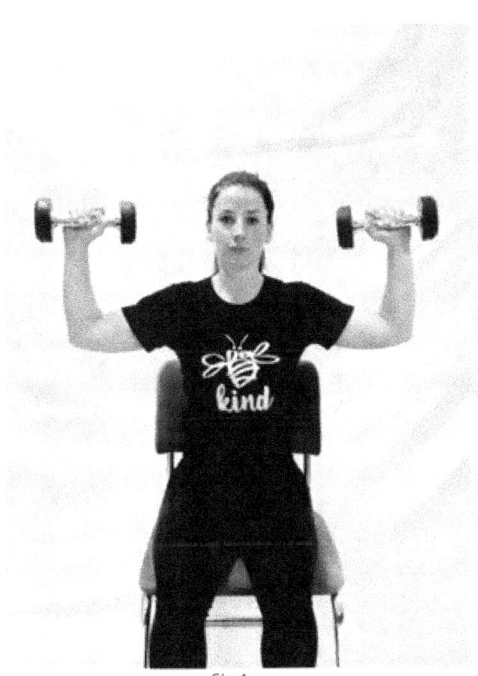

Fig 1

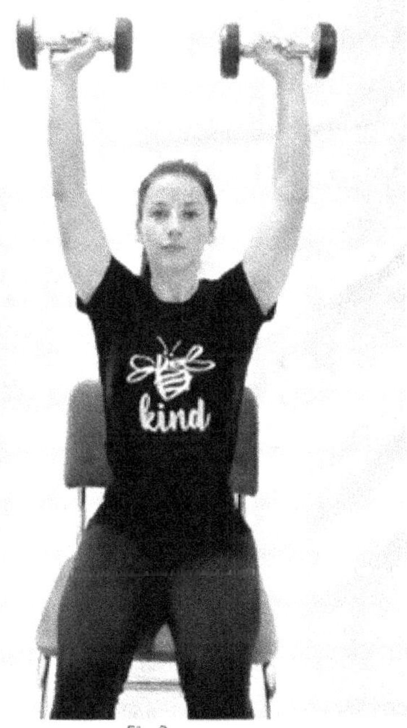

Fig 2

Lateral Raises

- Sit on a chair with your feet on the floor just over shoulder width apart and your back straight, looking straight ahead.
- Keep your arms by your side with a slight bend in your elbow holding your weights.
- Bring the arms up until they are parallel with the floor ensuring your hands do not go higher than your elbows at any time.
- Slowly lower the weight back to the start position.
- Tempo 1-2-3.

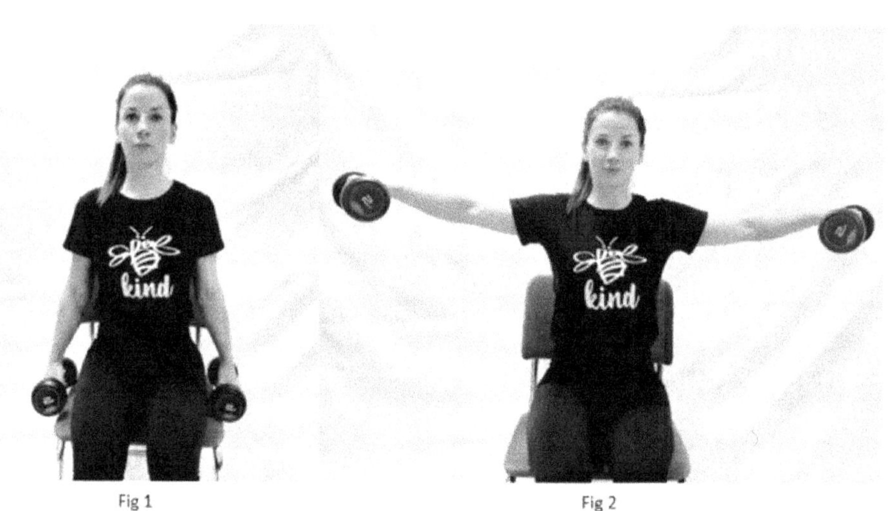

Fig 1   Fig 2

Bicep Curls

- Sit on a chair with your feet on the floor just over shoulder width apart and your back straight, looking straight ahead.
- Keep your arms by your side with a slight bend in your elbow holding your weights.
- Raise your hands up bending at the elbow, at the same time turn the palms of your hands to face upwards.
- Slowly lower back to the start position.
- Tempo 1-2-3.

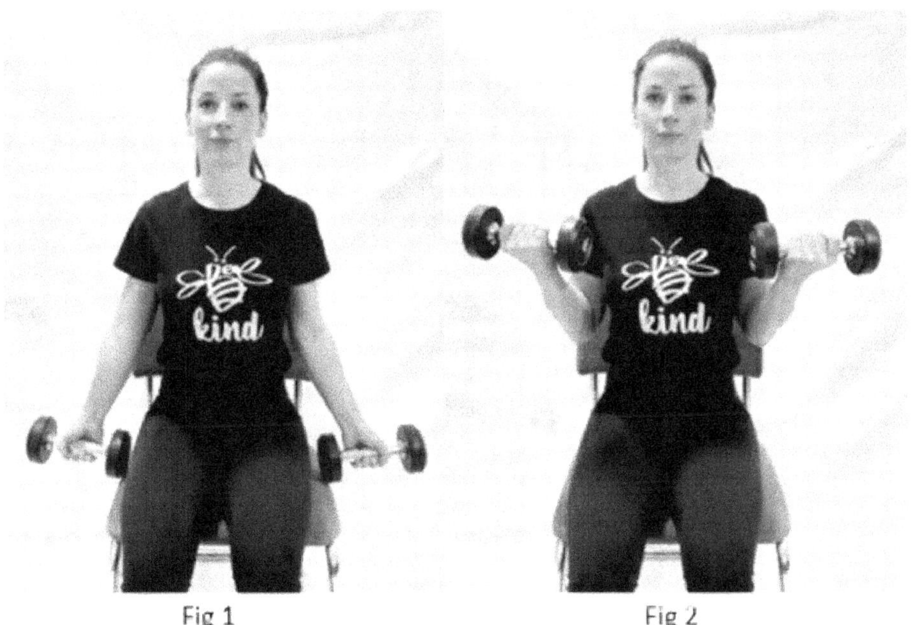

Fig 1   Fig 2

Chair Dips

- Use a chair or a step to place your hands on behind your body, keep your torso straight and have a 90degrees bend in your knees.
- keep both feet on the floor about shoulder width apart to ensure you have a good base of support.
- Slowly lower yourself by bending your elbows to 90 degrees or until your buttocks are close to the floor, straighten the elbows to bring yourself back up to the start position.
- Tempo 1-2-2.

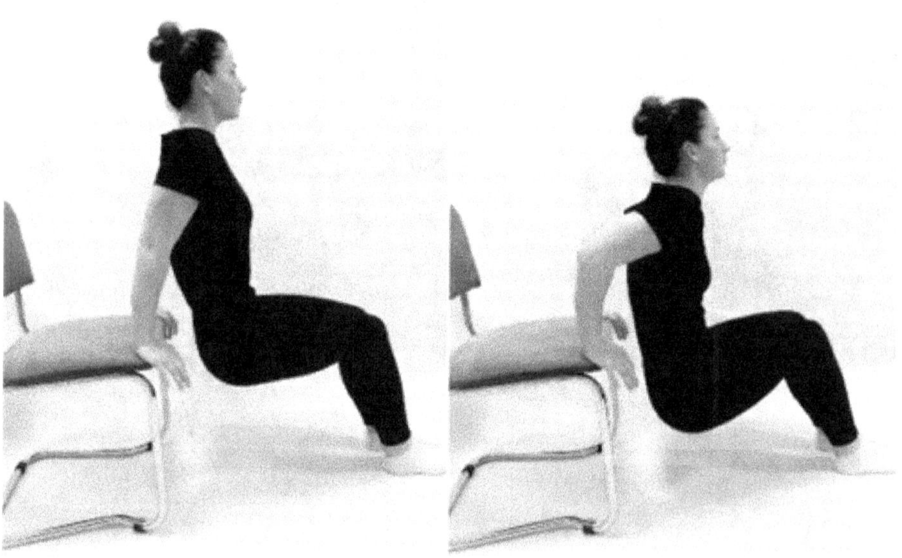

Fig 1   Fig 2

Upright Rows

- Stand with your feet on the floor just over shoulder width apart, a slight bend in your knees with your buttocks tensed and your back straight, looking straight ahead.
- Hold your small weights in each hand at the front of your hips.
- Pull your elbows up high so that they are above your shoulders keeping the weights to your front.
- Slowly go back to the start position.
- Do up to 15 repetitions 3-4 times.

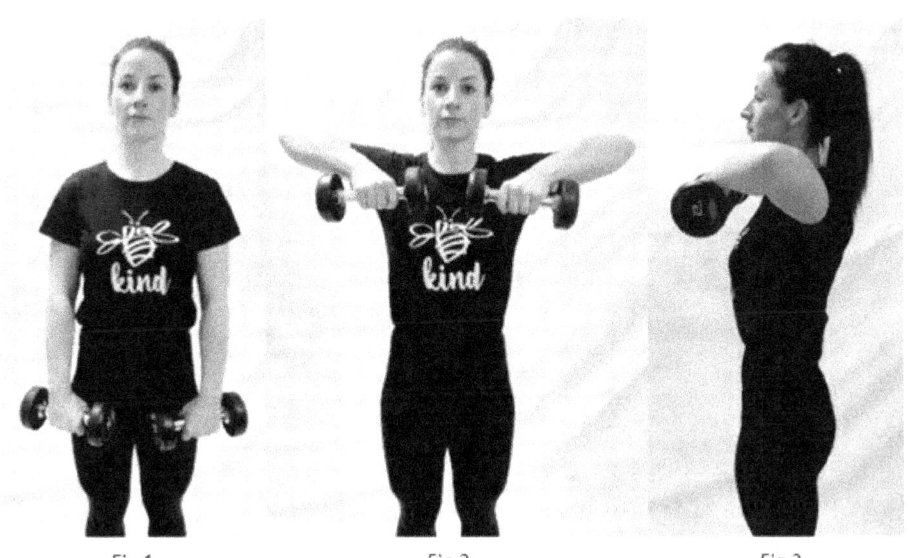

Fig 1   Fig 2   Fig 3

Bent Over Rows

- Stand with your feet on the floor just over shoulder width apart, a slight bend in your knees, bending over at the hips to a 45degree angle with your back straight, looking straight ahead.
- Have your arms hanging straight down in front of your holding your weights or resistance band.
- Pull the weights up to your sides ensuring your elbows come up higher that your back.
- Slowly lower back to the start position.
- Do up to 15 repetitions 3-4 times.

Dumbbell Variant

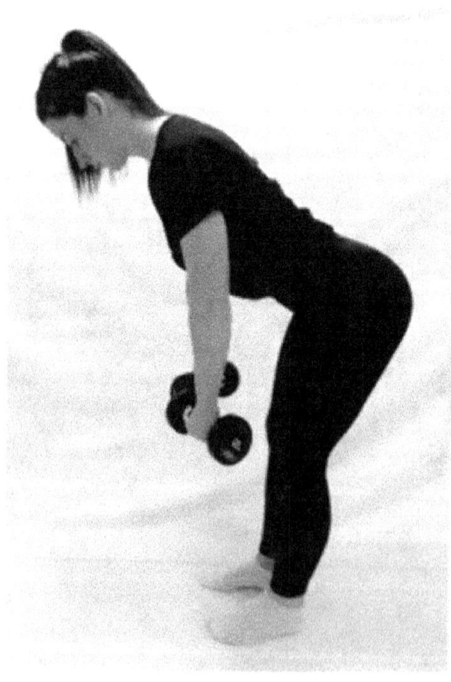

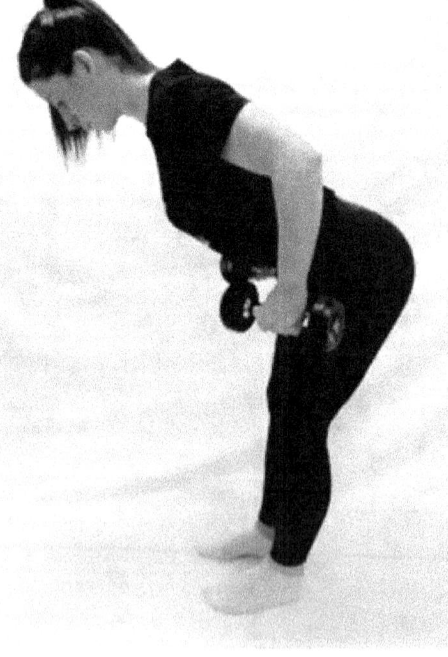

Fig 1Fig 2

Resistance Band Variant

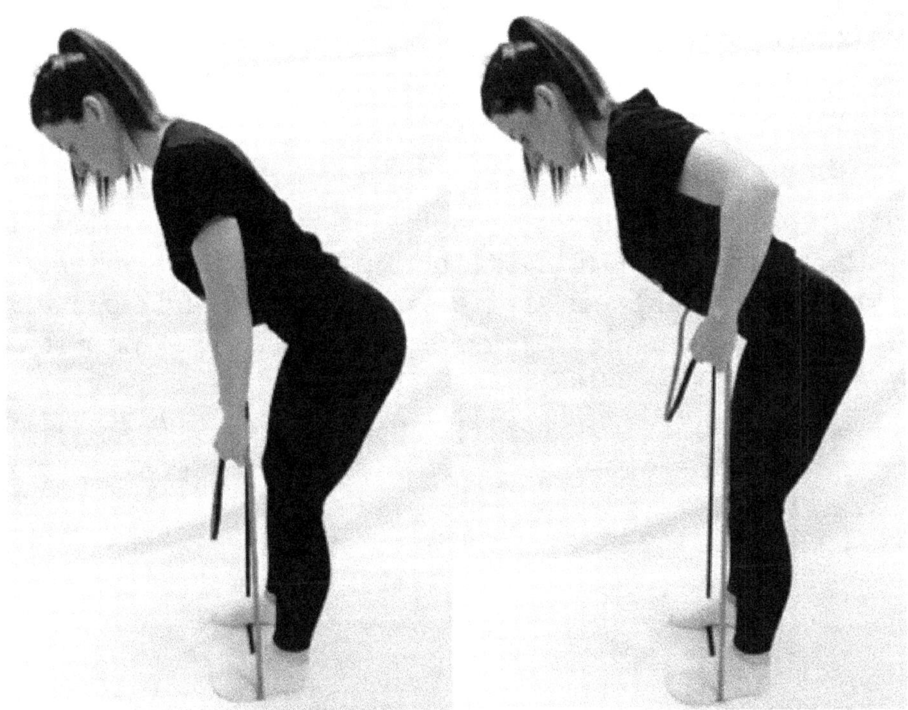

Fig 3   Fig 4

Cardiovascular Exercise

Running or Jogging

As with all exercise during pregnancy you should not increase your pre pregnancy levels however if you were running before you are fine to continue with your normal running routine unless directed to do otherwise by a medical professional of course.

Brisk Walking

Walking is an easy to do and beneficial way of exercising. It can be incorporated into your daily routine. Why not try 30 minutes every morning to start your day.

Non-Impact

Non-impact cardiovascular exercise is a great way to get your heart rate up and keep fit and can be done on a static exercise bike or another machine such as a cross trainer. It is useful especially if you are experiencing joint or muscle pain when walking or running.

This page has been intentionally left blank.

Don't have access to a machine? No problem try these.

Walk Outs

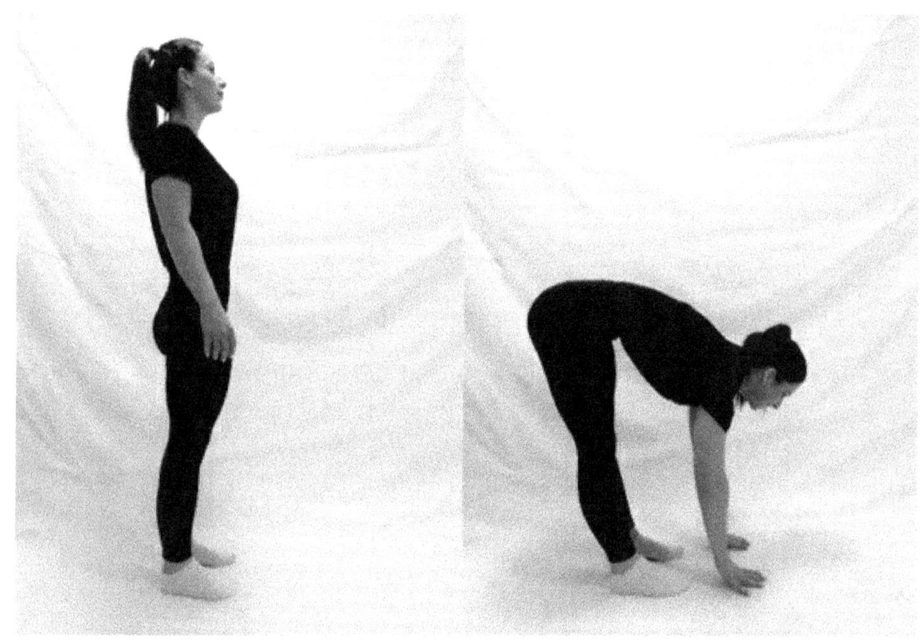

Fig 1   Fig 2

Walk Outs Continued...

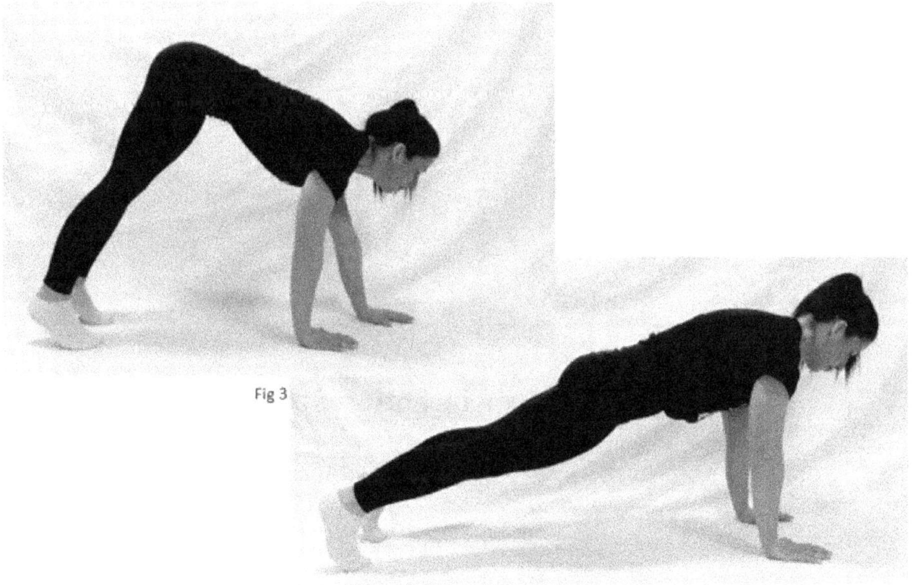

Fig 3

Fig 4

This page has been intentionally left blank.

CHAPTER 4 – EXERCISE POST PREGNANCY

TVA Activation

- Lay flat on your back with your knees bent and your feet about shoulder width apart.
- Feel for the two bony notches at the front of your hips. Once you have found those feel approximately 2 inches in and 2 inches down and you will feel a small ridge of muscle on each side. This is your TVA (transverse abdominus).
- Imagine your belly button is a zip and you want to zip it up and in towards your spine.
- Blow out the air and tense your stomach muscles at the same time.
- Hold your stomach muscles tight!
- Imagine you are going to the toilet and want to stop mid-flow this will activate your pelvic floor.
- The two small muscle ridges should remain hard throughout the exercise.
- Hold for 6-10 seconds and then reset to the start position.
- Repeat this 6-10 times.

TVA Activation Continued...

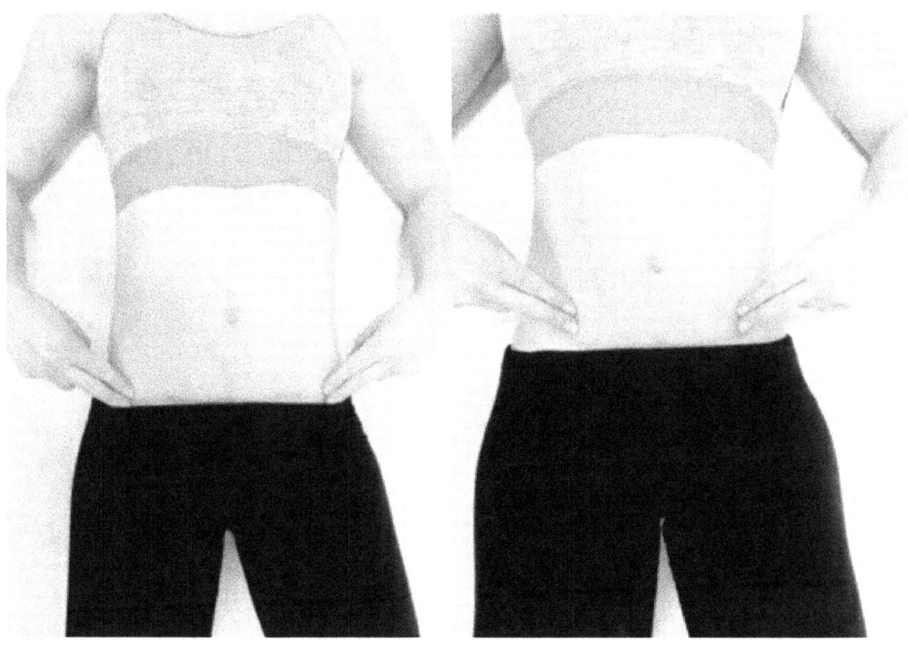

Single Leg Slides

- Do all the previous steps.
- When you are holding the position tensed, slowly slide one leg out.
- Your TVA should remain active the whole time you are sliding your leg out.
- Repeat with your other leg.
- Do 4-6 slides per leg.

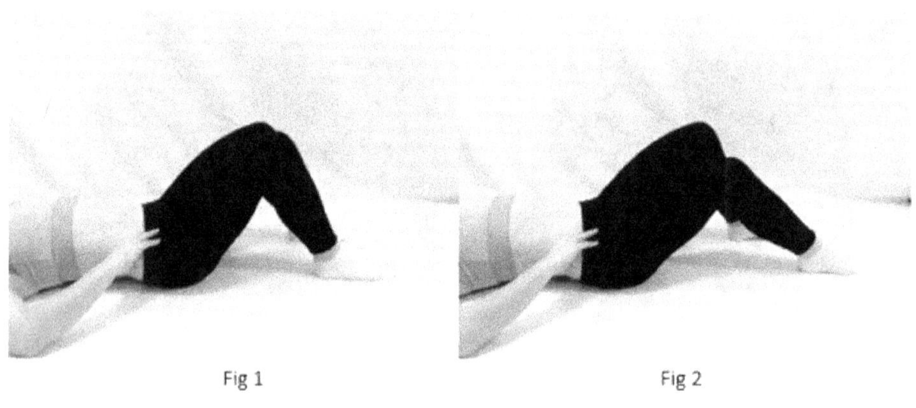

Fig 1   Fig 2

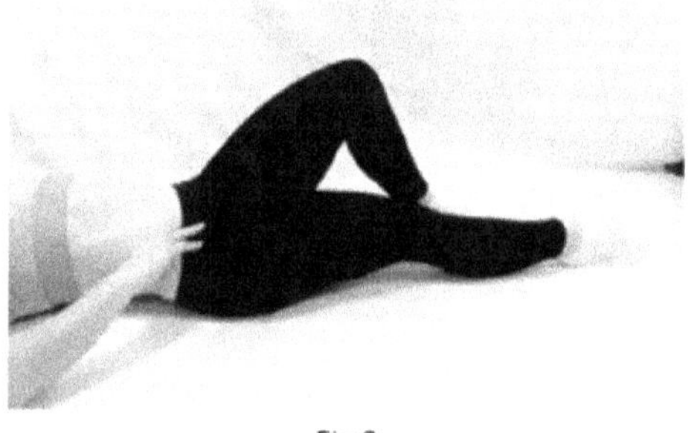

Fig 3

Arm Raises

- Do all the steps for TVA activation.
- When you are holding the position tensed, slowly raise one arm above your head as far back as you can go without changing the position of your spine.
- Your TVA should remain active the whole time you are raising your arm.
- Repeat with your other arm.
- Do 4-6 raises per arm.

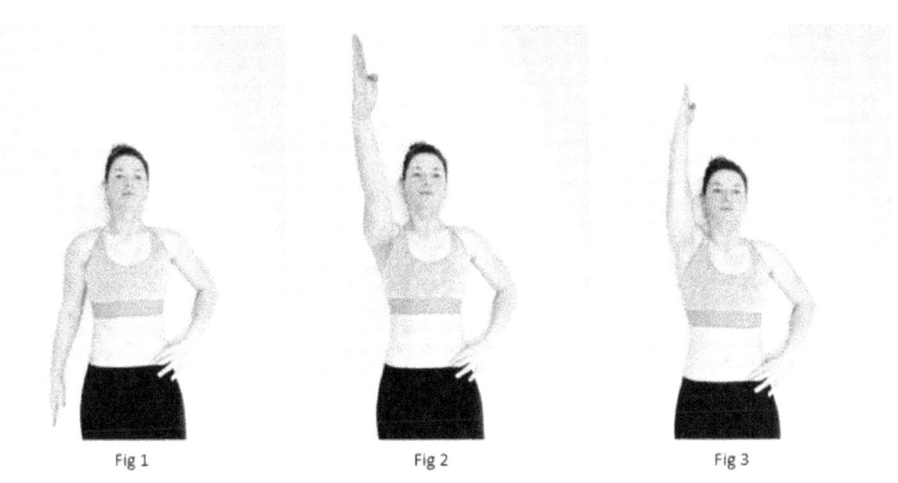

Fig 1   Fig 2   Fig 3

Dead Bugs

- Do all the previous steps for TVA activation.
- When you are holding the position tensed, slowly raise one arm above your head as far back as you can go without changing the position of your spine, at the same time slide the opposite leg out (for example your right arm and your left leg).
- Your TVA should remain active the whole time you are completing the movement.
- Repeat with the alternate side.
- Do 4-6 times per arm/leg.
- Tempo 2-1-2.

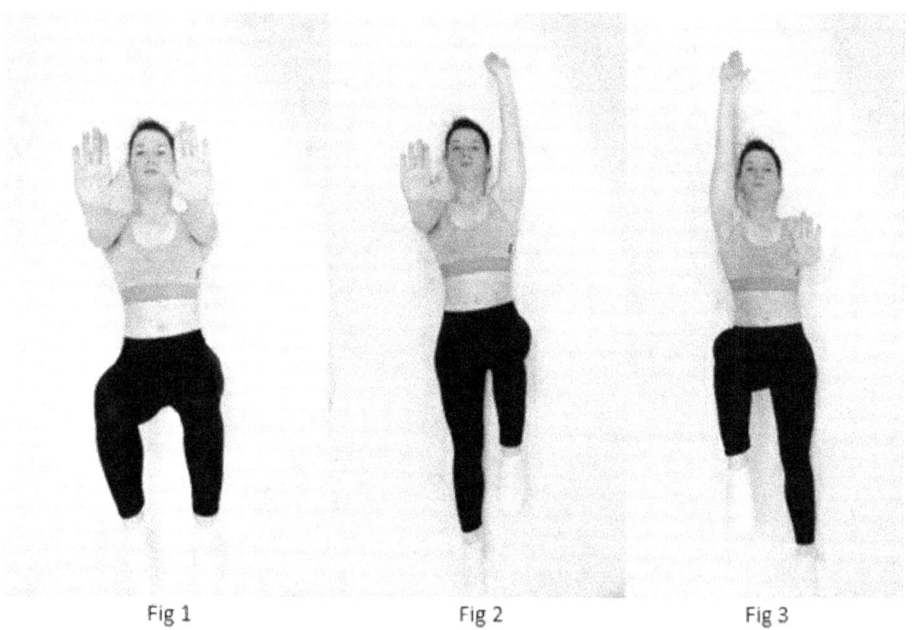

Fig 1   Fig 2   Fig 3

Dead Bugs Continued...

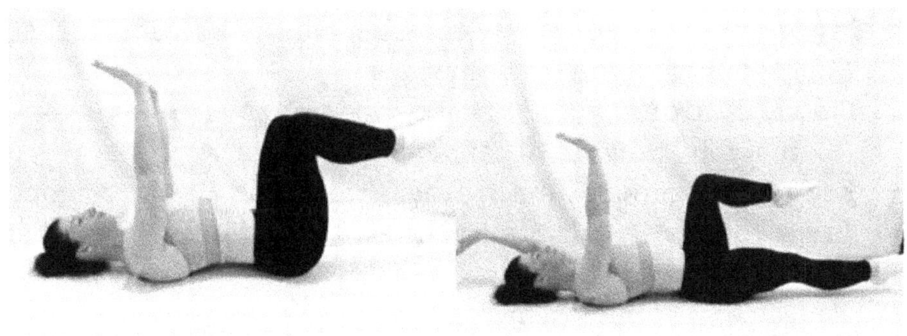

Fig 4

Fig 5

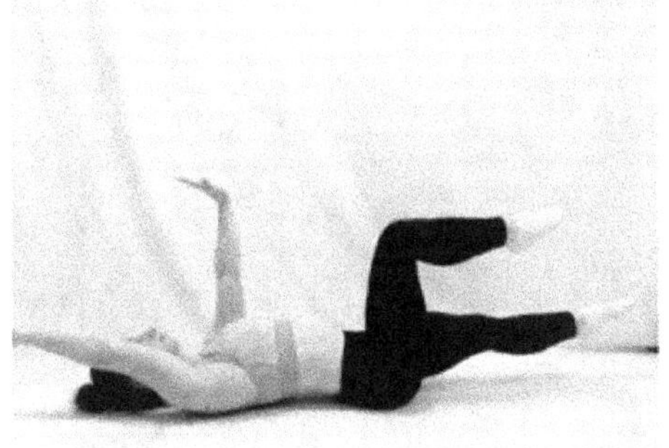

Fig 6

Knee Drops

- Lay on your back with your knees bent and your feet together, keep your hands out to your sides.
- Slowly drop one of your knees to one side to as low as is comfortable, keeping the other bent at 90 degrees.
- Keep your feet next to each other throughout the movement.
- Bring your knee back up to the centre and lower the other knee to the side.
- Repeat 10-15 times each side.
- Tempo 2-1-2.

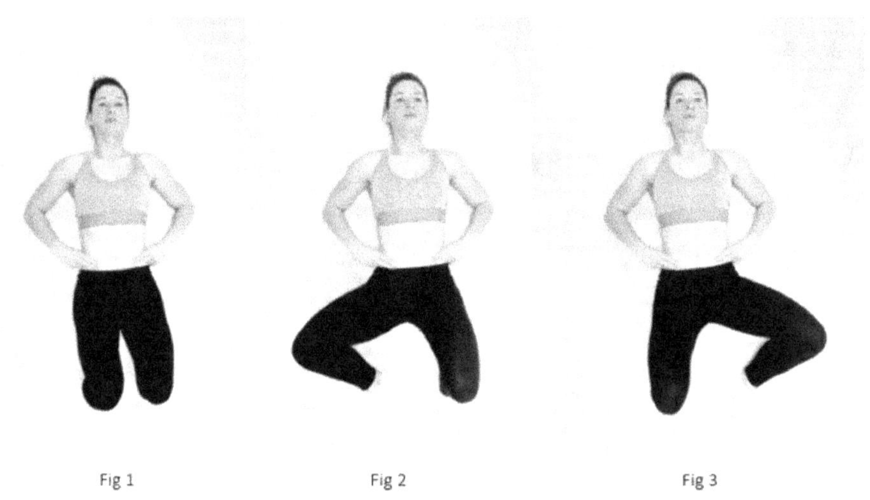

Fig 1   Fig 2   Fig 3

Single Leg Slide – Move out to the side

- Do all the steps to activate your TVA.
- When you are holding the position tensed, slowly slide one leg out and then to the side at roughly a 45 degrees angle to your body.
- Your TVA should remain active the whole time you are sliding your leg out.
- Repeat with your other leg.
- Do 4-6 slides per leg.
- Tempo 2-1-2.

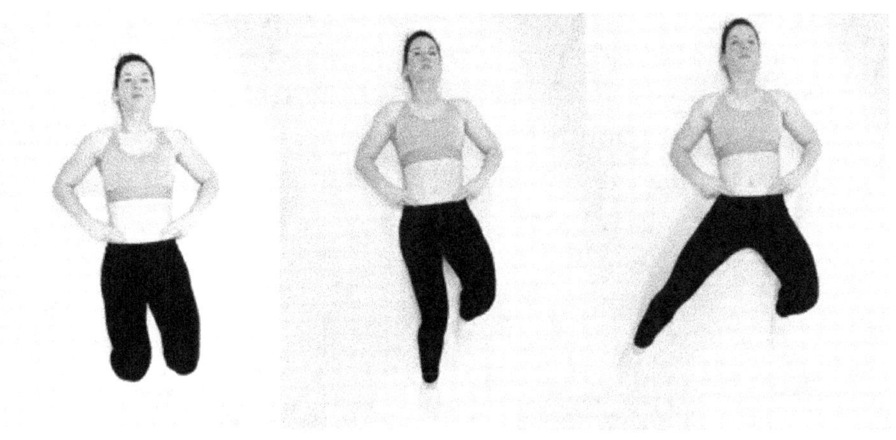

4 Point kneeling Flex and Vacuum

- Get onto all fours on a comfortable surface with knees under your hips, hands under your shoulders, with fingers facing forward and abdominals lifted to keep your spine neutral.
- Pull your stomach muscles in and raise your back upwards, curling the trunk and allowing your head to relax gently moving forward, putting your chin to your chest. Keep a slight bend in your elbows.
- Hold for a few seconds then slowly return to the start position.
- Ensure you do not arch your back: it should always return to a straight/neutral position.
- Do this slowly 10 times, moving your back carefully but ensuring your abdominals are working. Your back should remain comfortable throughout the movement.
- Tempo 0.5 -2-1.

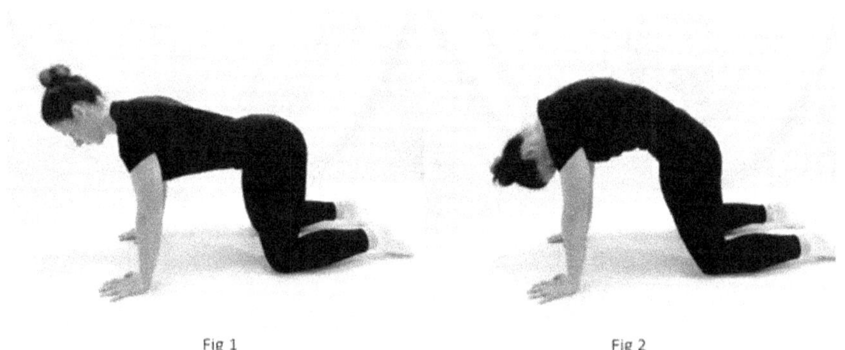

Fig 1   Fig 2

Pelvic Tilts
- Stand with your shoulders and buttocks against a wall or laying on a flat surface.
- Have a slight bend in your knees.
- Pull your belly button towards your spine (as if doing a zip up) so that your back flattens against the wall or floor: hold for four seconds then release.
- Repeat up to 10 times.

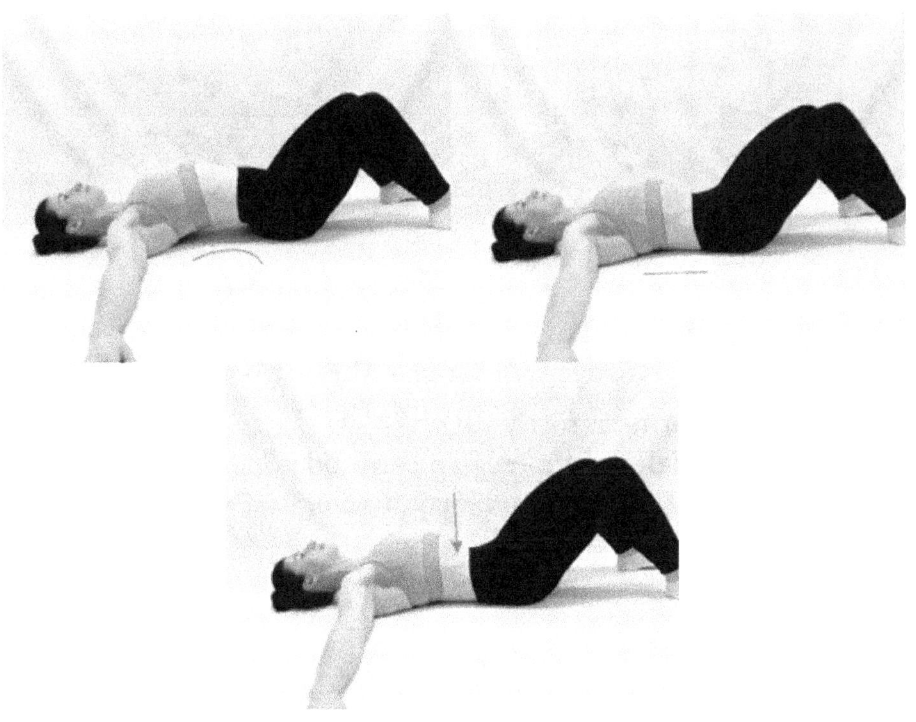

Bum Bridges

- Lay on your back with your hands by your sides and your feet together about 6 inches from your buttocks.
- Raise your hips up until your knees, hips and shoulders are in line, squeeze your buttocks hard and then lower.
- Tempo 1-3-2.

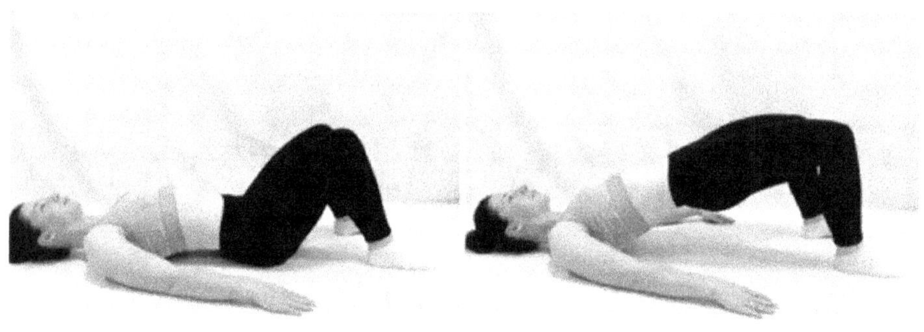

Fig 1   Fig 2

As you become stronger try some of these progressions:

- Put your arms across your chest.
- Wrap a small resistance band around your thighs.
- Squeeze a football between your thighs.
- Increase the tempo.
- Hold for time instead of repetitions.

Single Leg Bum Bridges

- Lay on your back with your hands by your sides and your feet together about 6 inches from your buttocks.
- Straighten one leg completely, ensuring your thighs stay in line and your knees stay together.
- Raise your hips up until your knees, hips and shoulders are in line, squeeze the buttock of the leg that is bent and then slowly lower.
- Do 10 repetitions of 3-4 times on each leg.
- Tempo 1-3-2.

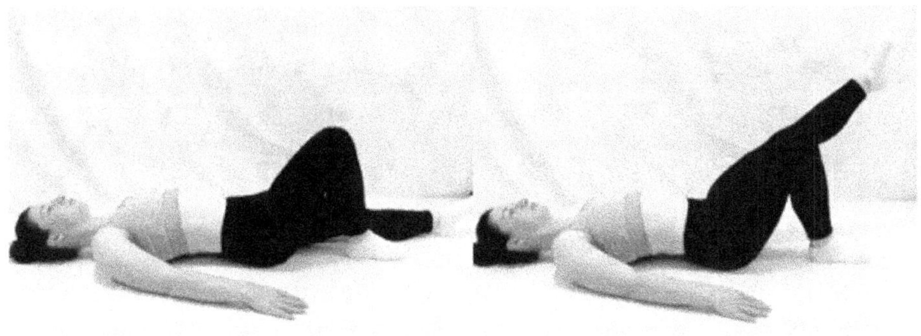

Fig 1   Fig 2

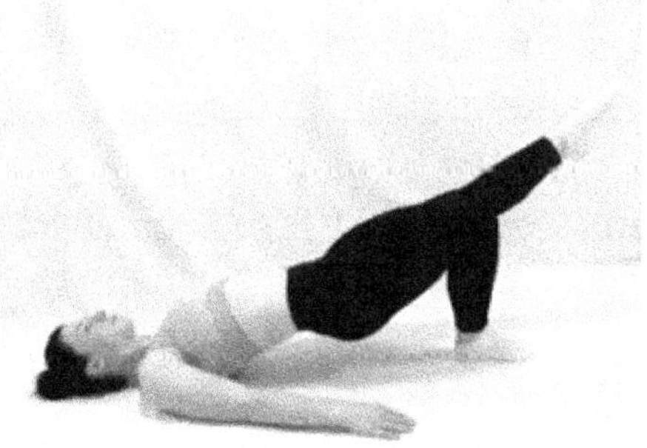

Fig 3

Plank

- Lay on your front then put your weight onto your forearms and toes so your whole body is off the floor apart from those body parts.
- Keep your elbows directly beneath your shoulders and maintain a neutral spine by looking directly at the floor and squeezing your abdominals and buttocks.
- Hold for 10 seconds and then repeat up to 10 times.

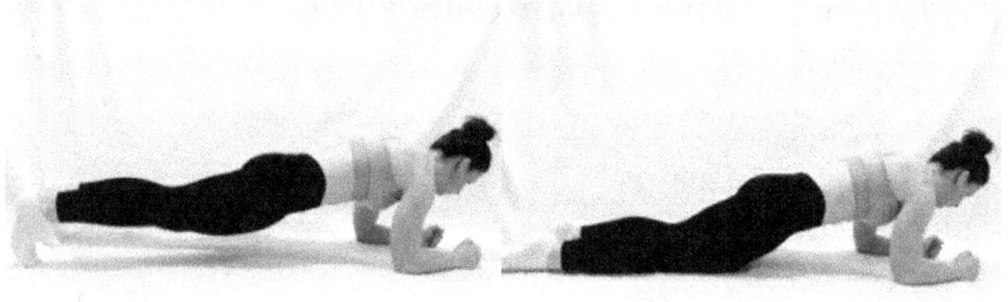

When you feel confident enough try making it interesting with these progressions:

- Increase the time.
- Lift one foot off the floor.
- Put your feet on a slightly unstable surface like a football or rolled up towel.
- Widen your stance and lift one arm off the floor.

Side Plank

- Lay on your side with your weight on one forearm, keep your knees bent and your legs together.
- Keep your lower leg and feet on the floor for support.
- Place your free arm down the side of your body and keep your shoulders in line with each other.
- To progress the exercise, straighten your legs and put your weight through the side of for feet.
- You should keep looking straight ahead throughout.
- Hold for 10 seconds and then repeat on to 10 times on each side.

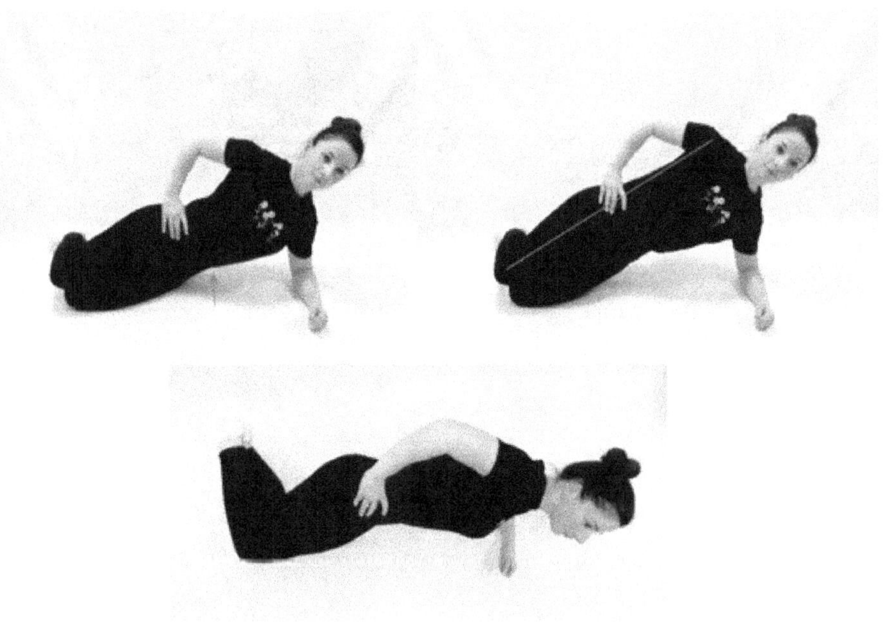

Side Plank Continued...

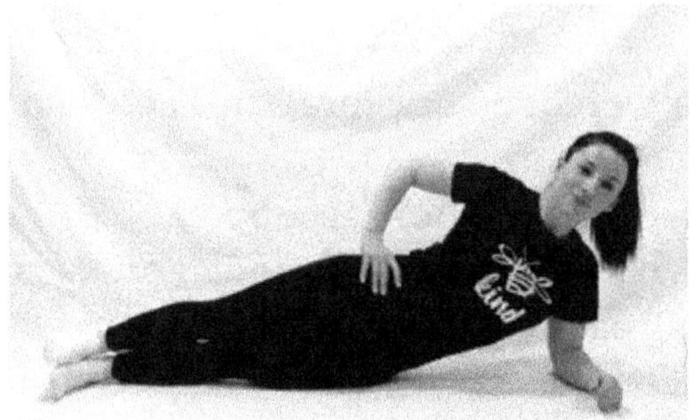

Fig 1

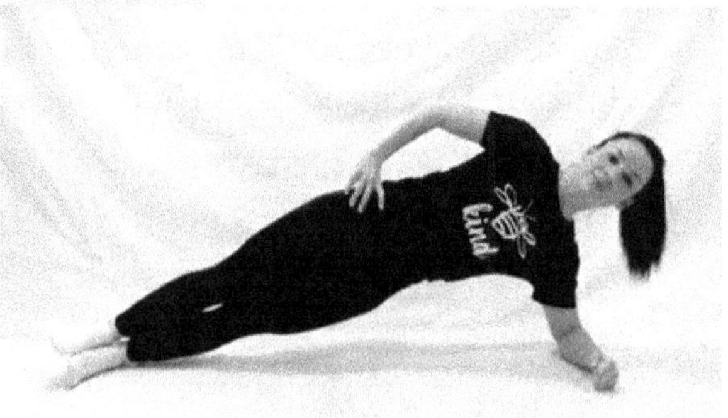

Fig 2

Clams

- Lie down on your side with both legs bent and your feet in line with your buttocks. Rest your head on your arm. Keep your free hand on your hip.
- Keeping your feet together slowly raise and lower your top knee.
- Your pelvis should remain in the same position throughout the movement and not move back and forth.
- Tempo 1-2-2.

   (Refer to page 31, Chapter 3 for demonstration pictures)

Hip Rotations

- Lie down on your side with both legs straight. Rest your head on your arm.
- Raise your upper leg and hold it in position.
- Rotate your hip forwards and backwards.
- Do up to 15 repetitions and repeat both side 3 times.
-   Tempo 0.5-0.5-0.5

   (Refer to pages 33-37, Chapter 3 for demonstration pictures)

Forwards Circles

- Lie down on your side with both legs straight. Rest your head on your arm.
- Raise your upper leg and hold it in position.
- Move your hip forwards in a circular motion imagining you are moving your foot around a football.
- Tempo 1 second to complete one full circle.

   (Refer to page 38, Chapter 3 for demonstration pictures)

Side Lying Abduction

- Lie down on your side with both legs straight. Rest your head on your arm.
- Lift your upper leg up and slightly backwards and then slowly lower it.
- Tempo 1-2-2.

(Refer to page 39, Chapter 3 for demonstration pictures)

Straight Leg Clam

- Lie down on your side with your bottom leg straight and your top leg bent with your foot in line with your buttocks. Rest your head on your arm.
- Keep your free hand on your hip.
- Keeping your foot on the floor slowly raise and lower your top knee.
- Your pelvis should remain in the same position throughout the movement and not move back and forth.
- Tempo 1-2-2.

(Refer to pages 42-43, Chapter 3 for demonstration pictures)

Feet Raised Clams

- Lie down on your side with both legs bent and your feet in line with your buttocks. Rest your head on your arm. Keep your free hand on your hip.
- Raise both feet off the floor.
- Keeping your feet together slowly raise and lower your top knee.
- Your pelvis should remain in the same position throughout the movement and not move back and forth.
- Tempo 1-2-2.

(Refer to page 32, Chapter 3 for demonstration pictures)

Running Man / Bicycle

- Lie down on your side with both legs bent and your feet in line with your buttocks. Rest your head on your arm.
- Keep your free hand on your hip.
- Keep your legs slightly apart.
- Keeping your bottom leg on the floor move your top leg in a running/cycling motion ensuring your legs remain parallel.
- Your pelvis should remain in the same position throughout the movement and not move back and forth.
- Tempo 2 to 3 seconds for one full repetition.

(Refer to pages 40 41, Chapter 3 for demonstration pictures)

Reverse Plank

-   Lay on your back with your elbows behind you and sup-
    ported on your forearms. (See picture).
-   Bent your knees slightly.
-   Lift your body up on the heels of both feet.
-   Move your feet closer to your body to make the exercise
    easier.
-   Tempo 0.5-1-0.5.

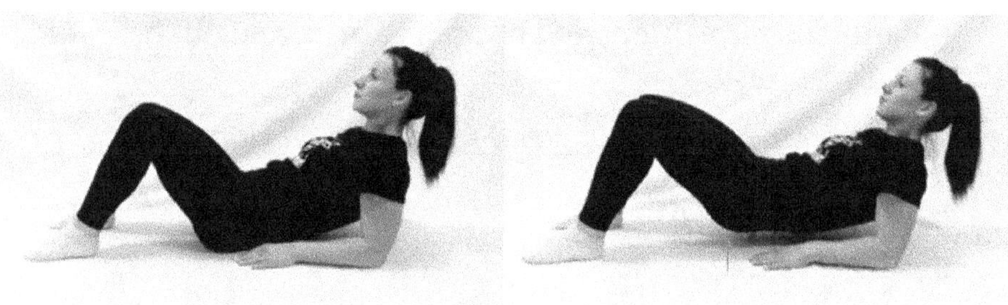

Fig 1   Fig 2

Push ups / Incline Push Ups

- Get down onto the floor and support your weight on your hands and toes. (See Fig 1).
- Keep the muscles of your core tensed and slowly lower your body towards the floor bending your elbows to 90 degrees.
- Straighten your arms to lift yourself back up.
- Try doing it on your knees at first until you get used to it. (See Fig 3 and Fig 4).
- Mix it up by doing incline push ups on a chair or raised surface.
- Tempo 1-0.5-0.5.

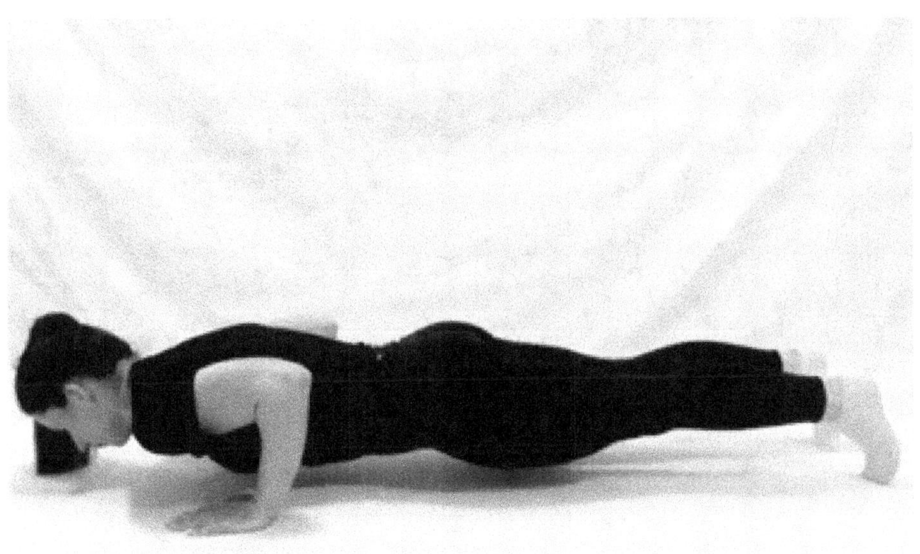

Fig 1

Push Ups Continued...

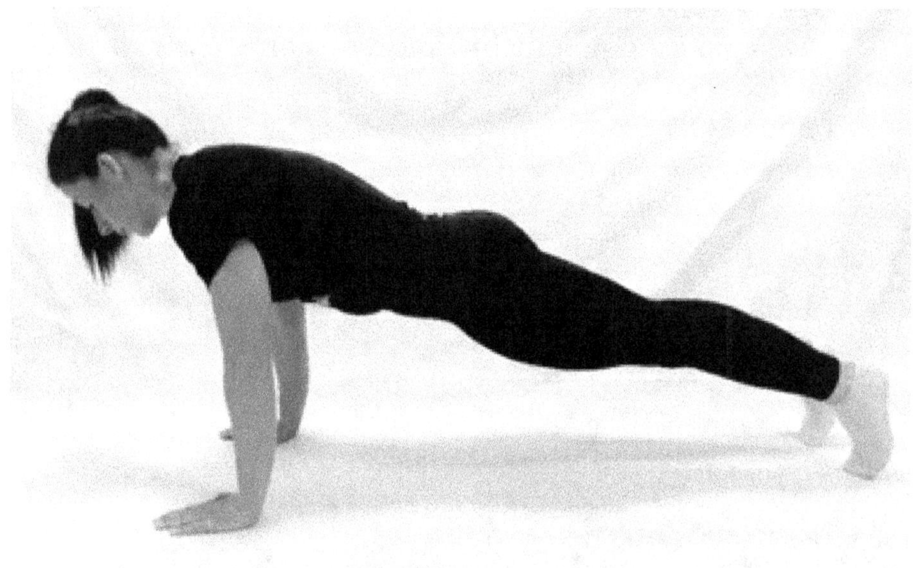

Fig 2

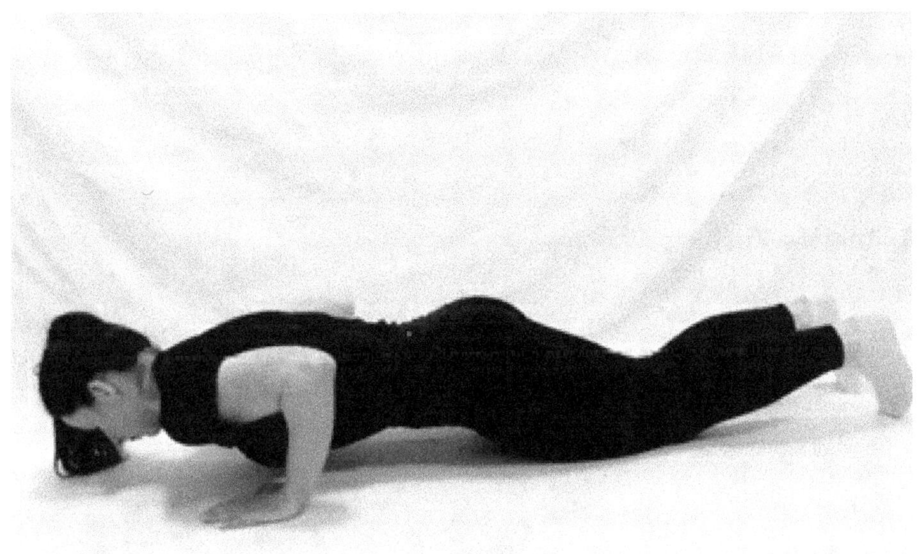

Fig 3

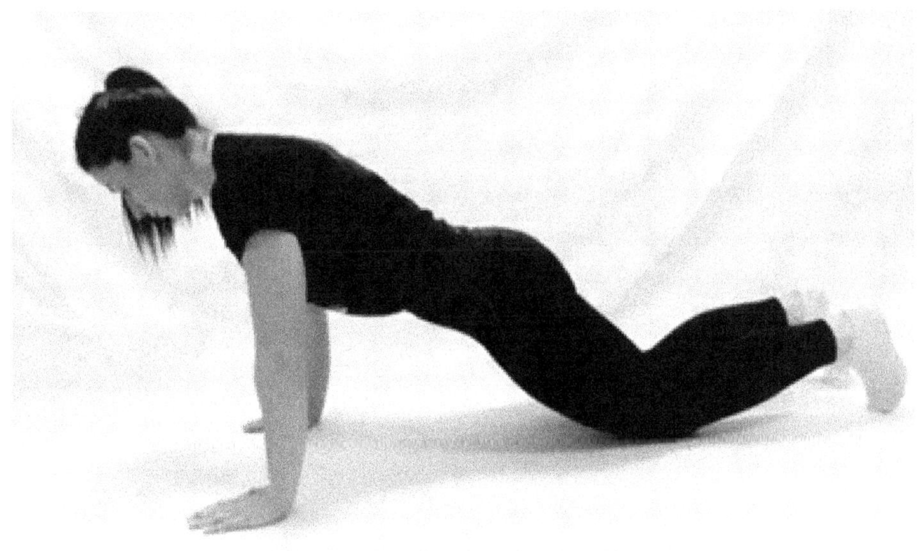

Fig 4

Incline Push Ups

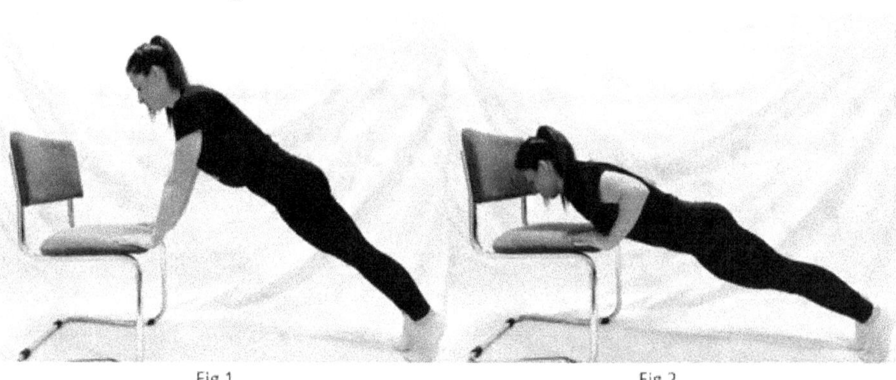

Fig 1   Fig 2

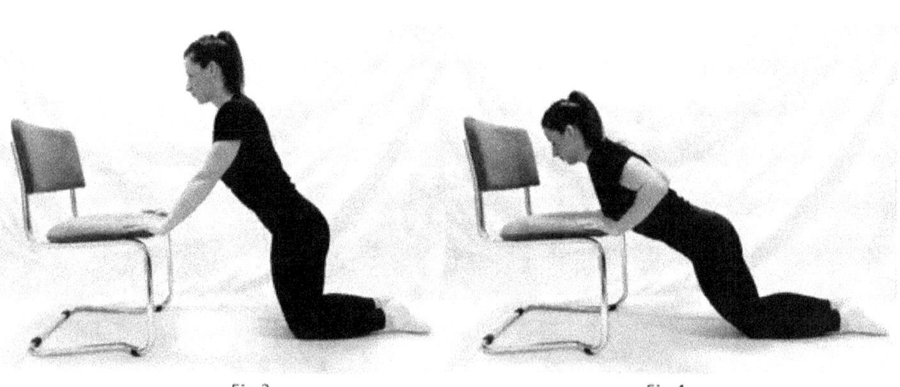

Fig 3   Fig 4

Hamstring Bridge

- Lay on your back with your hands by your sides and your feet together about 18 inches from your buttocks.
- Bring your toes off the floor so your weight will go through your heels.
- Raise your hips up until your knees, hips and shoulders are in line and then lower.
- You should feel this in the back of your thighs.
- To ease off a bit bring your heels closer to your buttocks.
- Tempo 0.5-1-1.

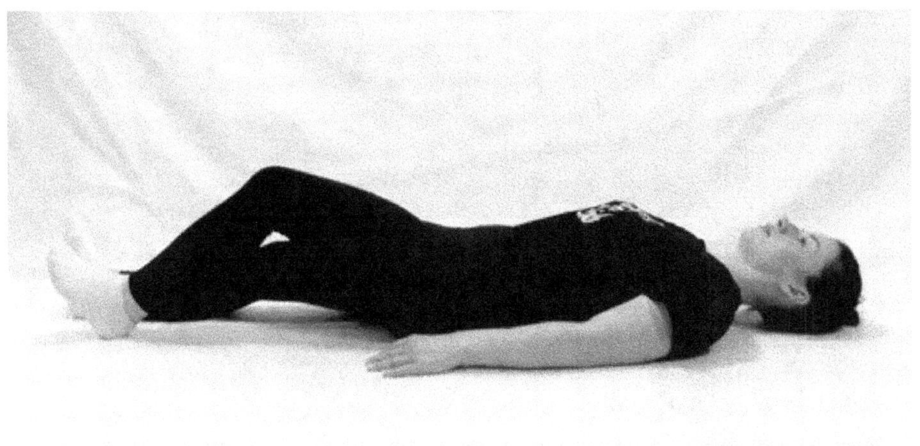

Fig 1

Hamstring Bridge Continued...

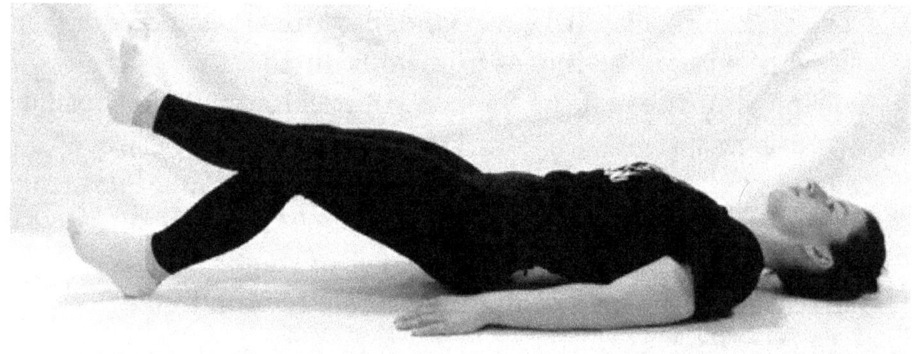

Fig 2

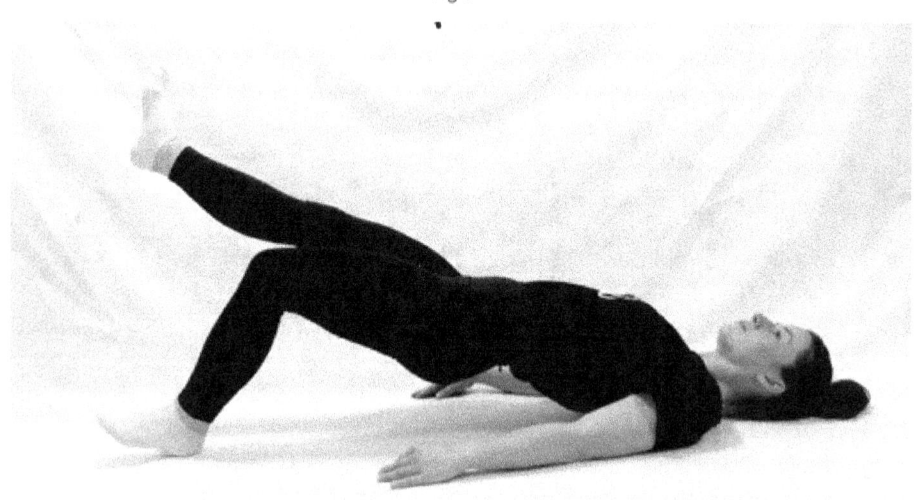

Fig 3

Myofascial Release

Myofascial release is a safe and effective technique that involves applying gentle sustained pressure to the myofascial connective tissue to eliminate pain and restore motion. In other words, putting pressure on your muscles to loosen them and allow tyou to move more freely.

Tools

Foam Roller and Ball

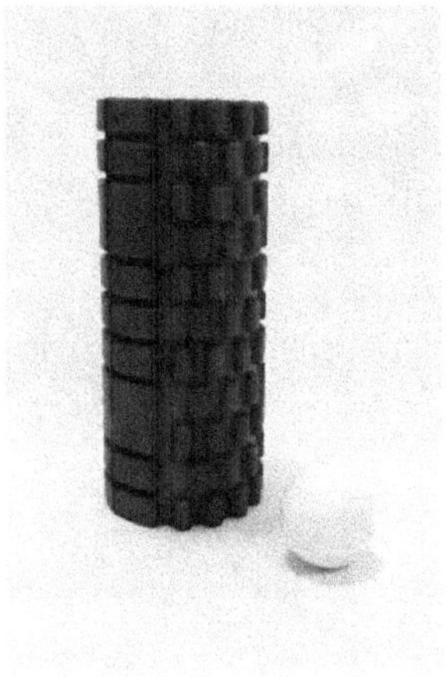

How

Begin rolling the desired part of your body on the foam roller. Ensuring the following points:

- Roll only on the fleshy parts of the major muscles.
- Support your weight to lessen discomfort.
- Ease in slowly, this will be uncomfortable at first.
- Avoid rolling over joints – This could cause injury!
- Do not roll over your spine.

Using a ball to roll will give a trigger point release effect and therefore it should be noted that this will cause more discomfort.

Foam and Ball Rolling the Legs

Calves

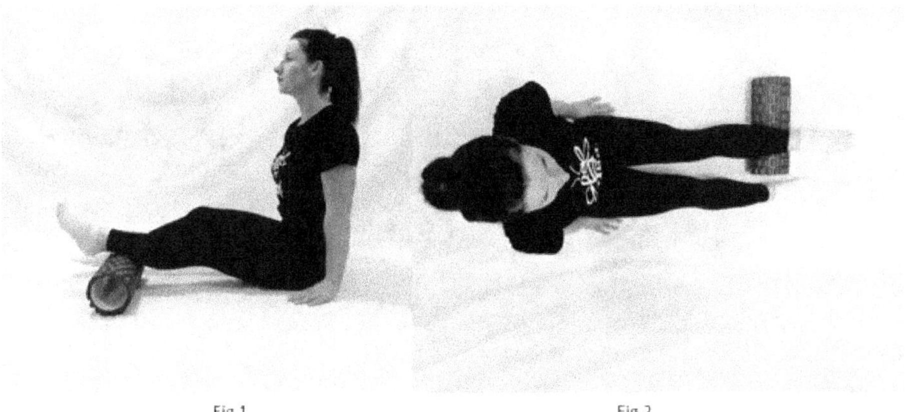

Fig 1   Fig 2

Hamstrings

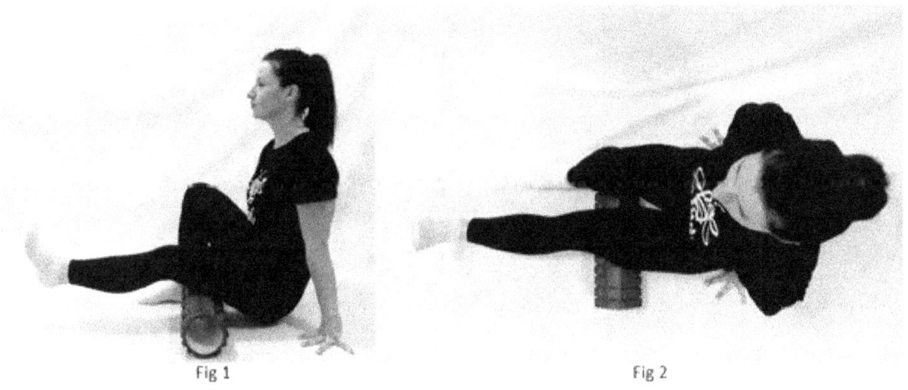

Fig 1   Fig 2

Quadriceps

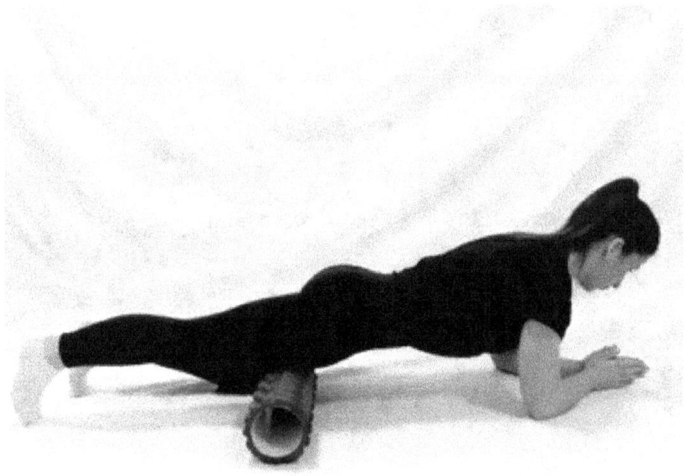

Fig 1

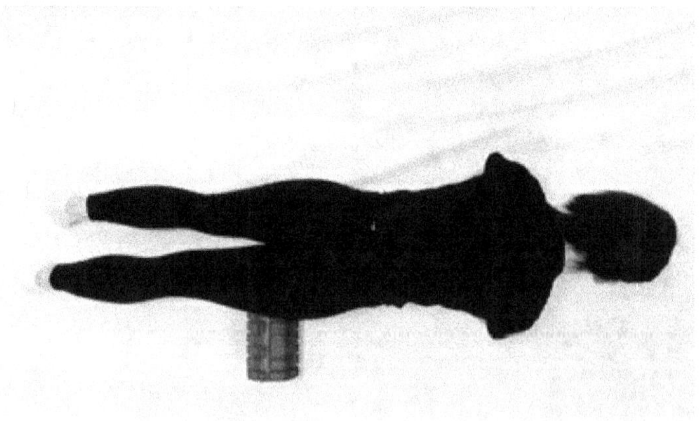

Fig 2

Buttocks

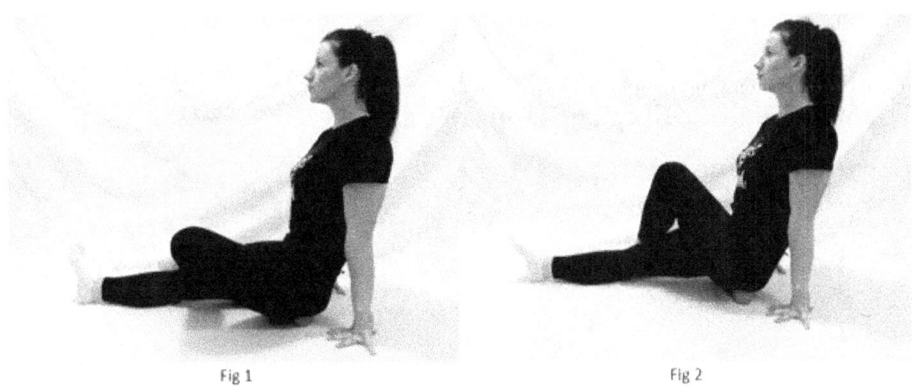

Fig 1   Fig 2

Foam and Ball Rolling the Upper Body

Deltoids (Shoulder Muscles)

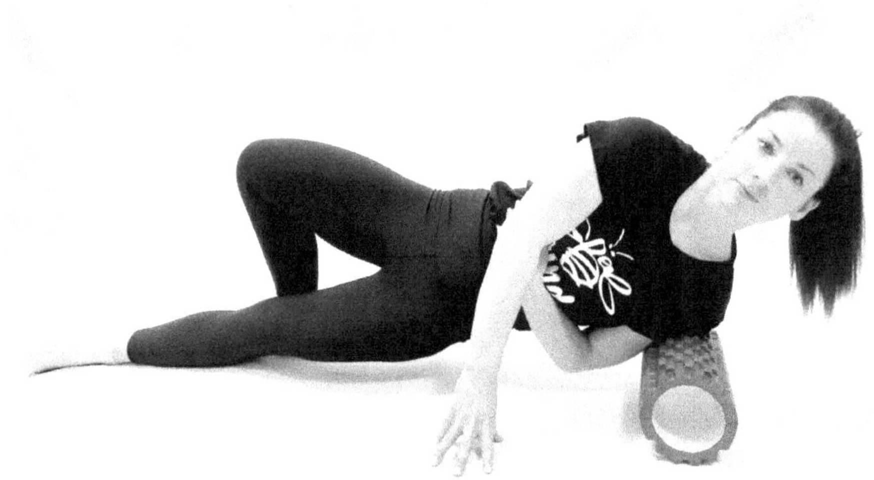

Pectorals (Chest Muscles)

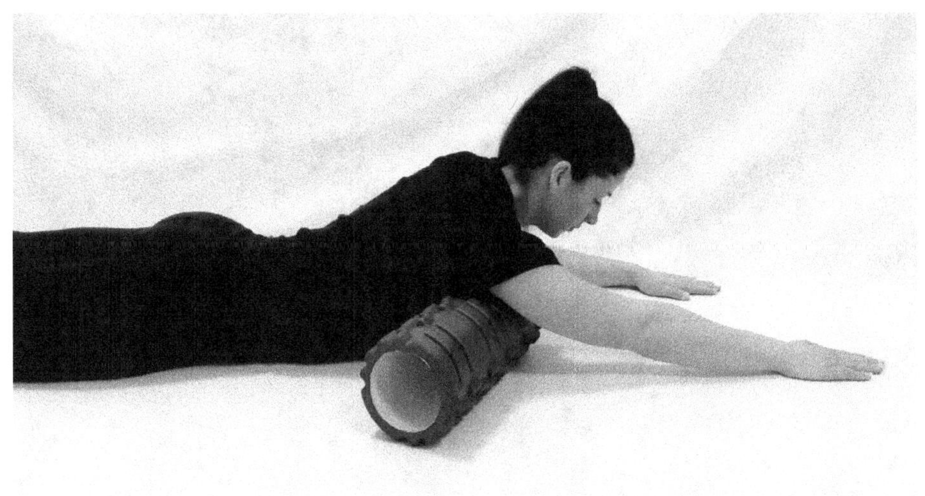

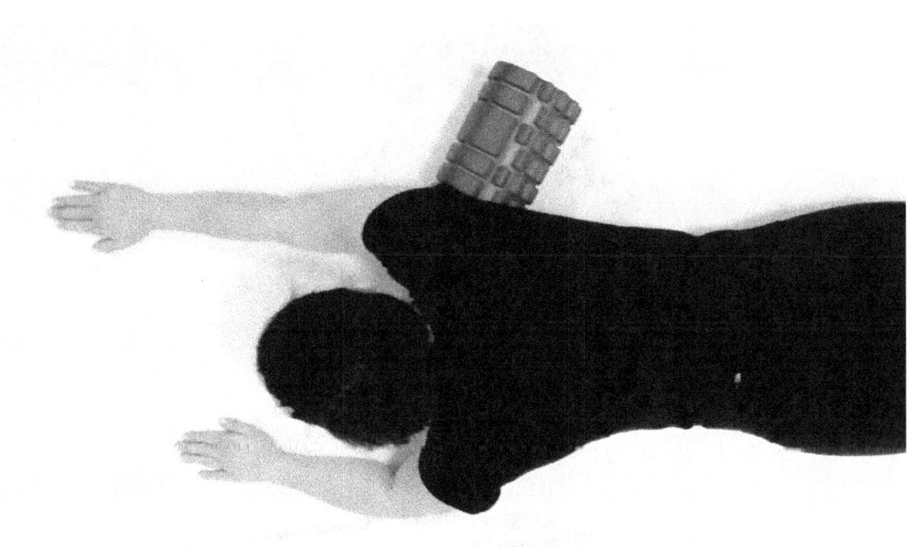

Biceps

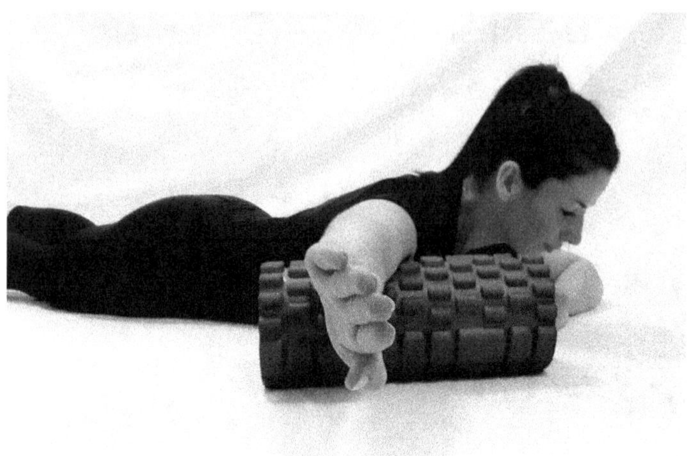

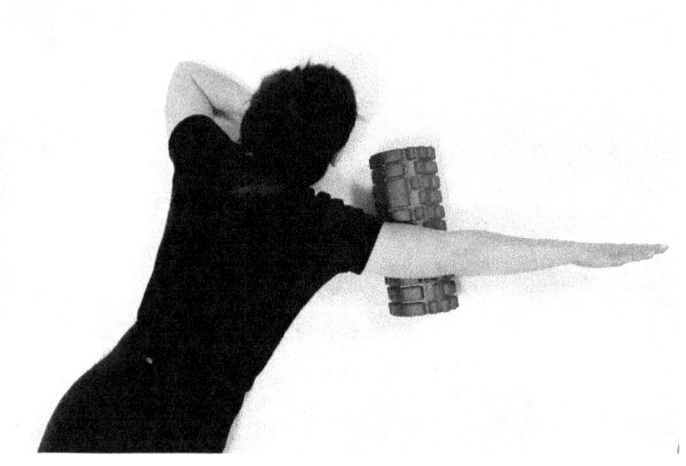

Latissimus Dorsi (Back Muscles)

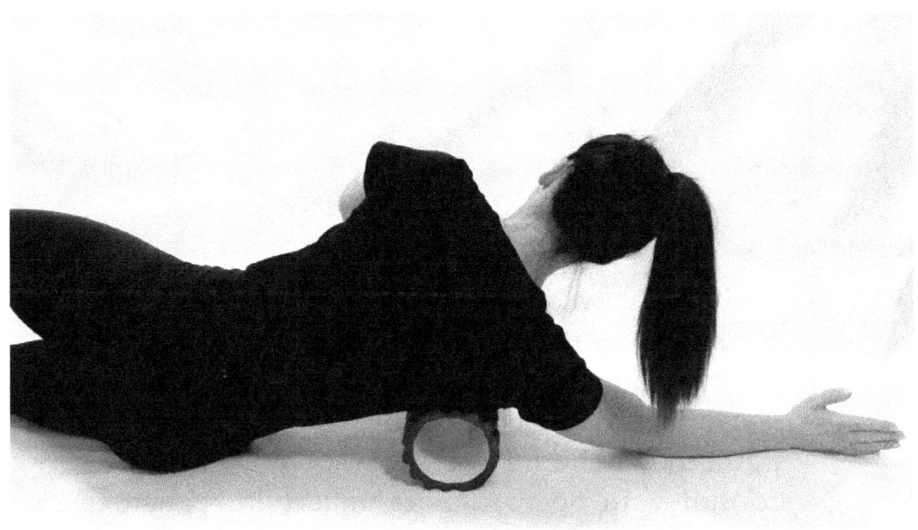

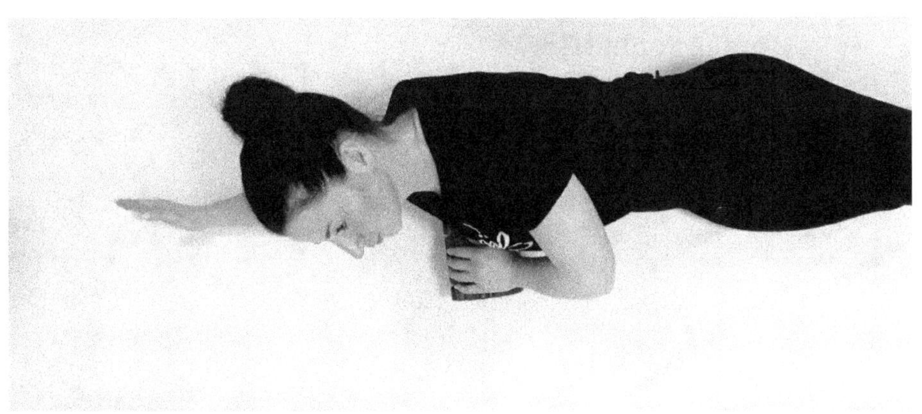

Notes

- During your second trimester calorie intake should increase by around 150Kcal per day. This should be from healthy sources such as fruit, vegetables, or lean meats.
- Dehydration can occur during your third trimester, so water intake should increase.
- Consult your doctor before undertaking any exercise plan.
- The content of this book is not intended nor should it be taken as medical advice or treatment.
- Model: Sophie Gray

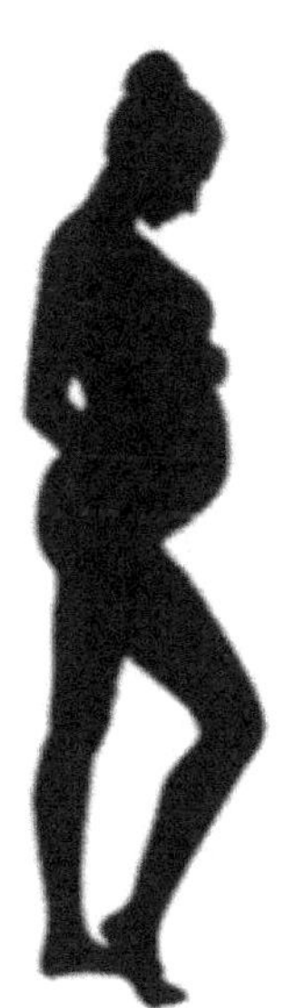